# My FIGHT with PD

A neurologist with Parkinson's disease

## David Blacker

Copyright © David Blacker, 2025
Published 2025 by the Book Reality Experience, an imprint of Leschenault Press, Leschenault, Western Australia

ISBN: 978-1-923454-12-5 - Paperback Edition
ISBN: 978-1-923454-13-2 - E-Book Edition

All rights reserved.

The right of David Blacker to be identified as author of this Work has been asserted by them in accordance with sections 77 and 78 of the Copyright, Designs and Patents Act 1988. No part of this publication may be reproduced, stored in retrieval systems, copied in any form or by any means, electronic, mechanical, photocopying, recording or otherwise transmitted without written permission from the publisher. You must not circulate this book in any format.

All source material has been fully acknowledged and used with permissions where applicable. Should you feel any material within is in breach of copyright please contact the publisher in the first instance.

*The author asserts that no Artificial Intelligence methods, techniques or tools have been used within the researching or production of this biography. Without in any way limiting the author's [and publisher's] exclusive rights under copyright, any use of this publication to "train" generative artificial intelligence (AI) technologies to generate text is expressly prohibited. The author reserves all rights to license uses of this work for generative AI training and development of machine learning language models.*

Cover Photo © Kirsten Blacker
Cover Design by Brittany Wilson | Brittwilsonart.com

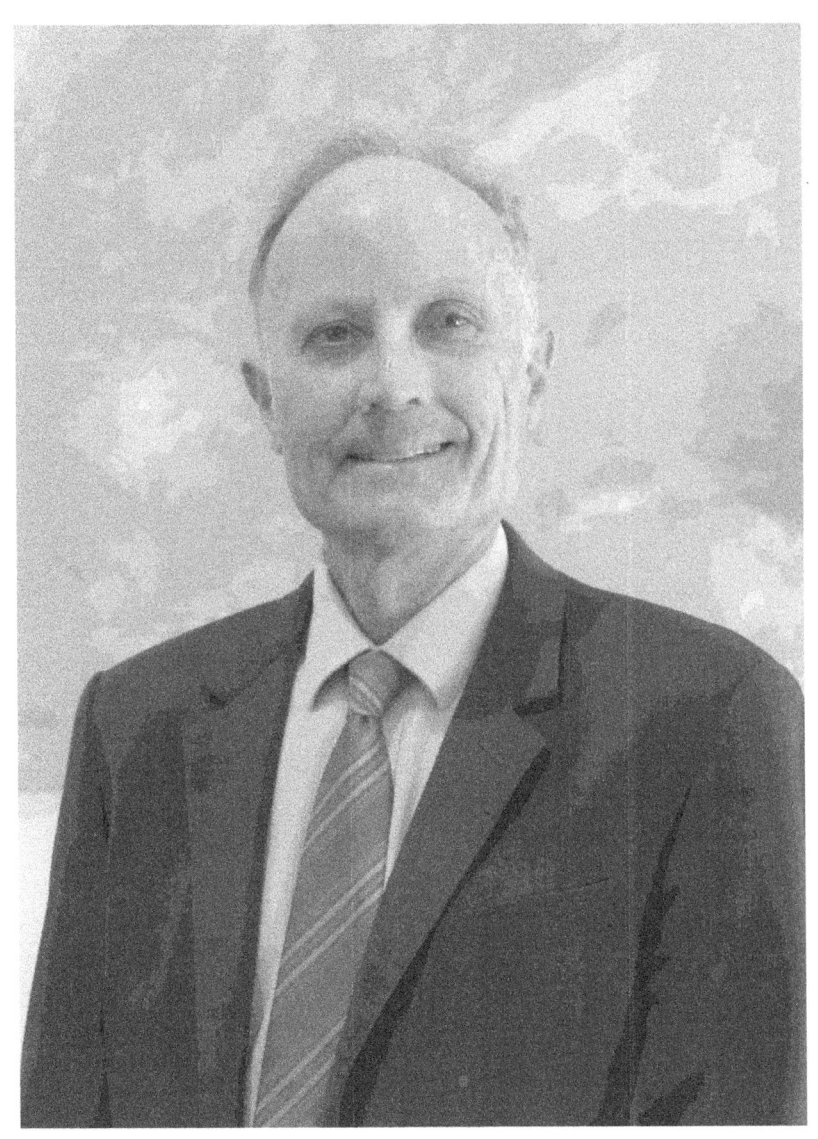

*The Author*

# Table of Contents

Notes on use of language ................................................................. i

Overview ........................................................................................ ii

Introduction ................................................................................... iii

BEFORE THE FIGHT

Who am I? - The early years ......................................................... 1

    Medical school ........................................................................... 1

    Early years of practice ................................................................ 2

    Neurology training ..................................................................... 4

    USA here we come .................................................................... 4

    Back to Australia ....................................................................... 5

    Losing the Minnesota lard ......................................................... 5

    My funky right foot ................................................................... 6

    Early experience with Parkinson's disease ................................ 7

    More symptoms emerge ............................................................ 9

    Impact on golf ......................................................................... 10

    Symptoms at work .................................................................. 11

    Time to start treatment ........................................................... 12

    Reaction to the diagnosis ........................................................ 16

'Coming out' – revealing the diagnosis ..................................................17

Hanging on for one tough year.......................................................19

Coming out 'big'..............................................................................22

# FIGHTing PD

Taking up the FIGHT against PD ..................................................27

Rai Fazio – a boxer joins the fight................................................28

Meeting Rai ....................................................................................31

Preparing FIGHT-PD.....................................................................32

FIGHT-PD works for me ...............................................................39

PD you can't see.............................................................................40

FIGHT PD begins – the early rounds............................................45

FIGHT-PD– the middle rounds ....................................................46

The final bell and beyond ..............................................................50

FIGHT-PD results ..........................................................................51

# The FIGHT is not over

FIGHT-PD – the documentary ......................................................57

UK Trip – COVID knocks me down..............................................57

Back to Perth .................................................................................63

Fatigue and depression..................................................................64

Changing gears and direction ......................................................66

2023 – a rollercoaster of events ....................................................68

PD when you can't see ..................................................................... 73

Too much of me on TV ...................................................................... 78

A brief escape ...................................................................................... 79

A new opponent .................................................................................. 80

100 days of cancer .............................................................................. 82

Fightback ............................................................................................. 89

Another trip ........................................................................................ 91

Taking stock and seeing the silver lining ........................................ 92

Three PD projects ............................................................................... 93

Yoga for PD ......................................................................................... 93

Support clinic for newly diagnosed PwP ........................................ 95

Fazio's PD Fighters ............................................................................. 96

The future – fighting on .................................................................... 98

Punching Paraquat .............................................................................. 99

Can the course of PD be altered? Studying the course of PD, and ways to favourably influence it ........................................................ 109

Finale (for now) ................................................................................. 113

Acknowledgments ............................................................................. 115

About the Author ............................................................................. 116

References ............................................................................................ 117

Dedicated to all those impacted by PD,
including their families and all those close to them.
I hope the story of my journey thus far
can help others on a similar path.

# Notes on use of language

The reader will note the title of this book uses the term Parkinson's Disease. However, in medical writing, there is a concerted attempt to reduce the use of eponyms (people's names) for disease[1]. Correct grammar does not require the use of the possessive apostrophe, unless the disease is named for someone who actually had it. Dr James Parkinson did not have Parkinson Disease (PD). I have determined to used Parkinson, with no apostrophe within the interior of this book. It gets tricky when reference is made to publications and organisations that have embedded the apostrophe in their title; in those instances, I have chosen to use it.

Where possible I have attempted to use the term person with Parkinson disease (PwP), rather than patient, since this is the preferred term for those who have the condition. In the context of clinical trials, the preferred term (suggested by many ethics committees) is participant.

There are some instances where I use the word patient, in reference to people I have cared for directly as their neurologist with PD, or other conditions. Some may view this as old fashioned, but I believe the term patient confers a sacrosanct relationship between patient and doctor that harks back to the Hippocratic Oath. To me, the term 'patient' automatically infers confidentiality, safe treatment and advocacy.

# Overview

This book has three sections. The first, 'Before the fight,' explains my personal and professional background and describes the emergence of PD symptoms, their impact on me, the diagnosis and early years of treatment. The second, 'FIGHTing PD' outlines how I have tackled my own PD, particularly through the use of exercise. I describe how I joined forces with Rai Fazio, former boxing champion, and a team of exercise scientists to create an exercise program based around non-contact boxing, which we named FIGHT-PD. The third, 'The FIGHT is not over,' describes my ongoing efforts to keep PD at bay from 2022 to 2024, in the face of a series of other illnesses. These included a bout of COVID-19, three eye operations, depression and prostate cancer. It was also the time during which I retired from clinical work. The section concludes with my rededication to exercise, adjustment of medications and reorganising of priorities, all of which helped to pull me back from acceleration of PD symptoms. I then outline three projects commenced during 2024, which had immediate impact for PwP: a specific clinic for newly diagnosed PwP, a program introducing yoga to PwP designed and run with my wife Kirsten, and my ongoing work with Rai bringing what we learned in FIGHT-PD to as many PwP as we can.

    I conclude by describing the issue of pesticides and the possible link to PD which captured a lot of my attention from the second half of 2024 onwards. However, I suspect my greatest opportunity to make a difference will continue to be using my rare position as a PwP and neurologist to help both groups understand each other more closely and enrich the clinical relationship.

# Introduction

In late 2018, I revealed to family, friends and colleagues that I have PD. This marked a change in the direction of my life and career. It has led me down a path I had never expected to pursue, but in many ways I was well prepared for. Curiously, my own experience with PD may have made my life more meaningful and fulfilling. As a neurologist and medical researcher who has PD, I have a unique opportunity to incorporate what I have experienced as a person with PD into research and treatment for others. This book describes my life story and the impact PD has had on me. Where possible, I try to provide some information about PD, as well as my perceptions and feelings. I hope this might benefit others with PD and their families.

The acronym FIGHT stands for Feasibility of Instituting Graduated High-intensity Training. This was a clinical feasibility trial of exercise using non-contact boxing that I developed with former boxing champion Rai Fazio and some prominent sports scientists. The experience of designing, undertaking, then having the trial published, has been one of the highlights of my career and occurred while I was coming to terms with retiring early from clinical practice due to the impact of PD and a series of other health issues. The power of exercise, positive attitude and the amazing support from my wife have helped me to continue to live well, and convinced me that these interventions when applied promptly and expertly, can alter the course of PD. It has also given me a second career advocating and fighting for the benefit of people with PD.

# BEFORE THE FIGHT

# Who am I? - The early years

I was born on 5 July 1968 in Bunbury, the largest town in Western Australia, outside the capital Perth. My father was a schoolteacher, my mother a housewife. My brother was born in 1971. Rural service was a big part of teaching in those days, so we were to move several times to small country towns.

We moved to Perth in 1978 because my parents preferred that Mark and I attend secondary school in the city. I did well at high school, probably related to being a voracious reader from a young age. During our time in the country, television reception was limited, but I had access to the whole school library.

In high school I recall reading Freud's *The Interpretation of Dreams* and was interested to learn that Freud made it a practice to eat salty olives just before bedtime in order to wake up thirsty in the middle of a dream, which he could then write down and interpret. By my mid-teens I was fascinated by the brain/mind interface, and continued to read about the topic during high school. I was also a sports nut, loving cricket, and golf, winning the state under-12 age group golf championships, and cutting my handicap to single figures and then later to 3 at university. I had a full and energetic high school experience, participating in sports, music, drama and debating. I graduated in 1985 and the following February commenced medical school at the University of Western Australia.

## Medical school

I can't recall a specific decision to study medicine. At high school, there seemed to be an assumption in that era that if you did well academically, you would go on to study medicine or law, or maybe engineering. Even though I was on the high school debating team, and could certainly construct a good argument quickly, there was no way I had any thoughts about studying law. I had also realised that my dreams of opening the batting for the Australian Cricket team, or playing professional golf, were not really feasible mainly because I wasn't good enough.

So I found myself at medical school. On the orientation day, we were taken on an extensive tour, which included the morgue. The pathology professor showed us a cadaver and asked us what may have been the cause of death. I immediately piped up, 'it could have been an aneurysm' as I'd heard about aneurysms on a popular television soap opera around that time, *The Young Doctors*. The professor seemed taken aback. 'Yes it was! You could get a job here one day young man.' And as a matter of fact I did.

A highlight of medical school was in May 1990, when I met my wife to be, Kirsten, during one of my earliest medical research projects. As part of the fifth-year course, we undertook a group project and my group was tasked with investigating passive cigarette exposure in non-smokers. To do this, we had to find venues where there was a lot of cigarette smoke and soon settled on the local bars; medical students were quite familiar with these. At one of these venues, Kirsten was enrolled as a participant in the study. Perhaps this fuelled my enthusiasm for medical research.

## Early years of practice

My intern year was at Sir Charles Gairdner Hospital (SCGH), a major teaching hospital in Perth, with over 600 patients. My first rotation was in general surgery. I quickly learnt how to be a young hospital doctor, but didn't find this job particularly fulfilling. One of my allocated tasks was to enter patient data into a computer data base for an audit. This was a new concept at the time, and I found it boring and frustrating; certainly not what I had pictured as doctoring. One day, while I was scrubbed in as a surgical assistant, I heard a noise behind me. I turned around and saw one of the theatre orderlies on the floor having a seizure. The surgeon seemed unconcerned by the emergency occurring a few meters away and so I instinctively rushed over to help, leaving the operation, in which my role was very minor. Thankfully, the orderly recovered after I found him to be hypoglycaemic, and treated him. This was a sign as to where my medical interests were gravitating.

My second term as an intern was in neurosurgery. This changed everything for me. Sir Charles Gairdner Hospital had a comprehensive neurosurgical service, covering an enormous geographic territory. The intern experience was rigorous, exceeding 100 hours per week, but I thrived because of the nature of the work. I still remember the thrill of seeing a live brain exposed during surgery. This was the organ I wanted to learn as much as possible about.

My next rotation was psychiatry. With my interest in the brain and mind, I had thought this was going to be my calling, but I soon realised that I felt out of place with hospital-based psychiatry practice and the more laid-back pace of the psychiatry wards. The leisurely 9 am starts with coffee and a meeting of the psychiatry team were in stark contrast to neurosurgery, where I'd usually done the ward round by then, ordered the CT scans for the day and started on my third coffee. My seniors on the psychiatry team thought I was a little 'hyped up.'

I completed my intern year, and then moved into a second year of resident medical officer rotations, which included a second term of neurosurgery. I had no clear plans to pursue a surgical career, but was keen to have another look at the brain, and no neurology rotations were available. In August, I took a short break to get married and honeymoon. By that time, Kirsten and I had been living together for a couple of years. In early 1994 I did my first rotation in neurology, and I immediately felt this was the area for me. Two terms of neurosurgery, and a term of psychiatry had provided a solid grounding in neuroscience. I liked how neurology seemed to fit nicely in between those two specialties. It gave me very good grounding for future consultations on patients from these areas. Neurosurgery might be regarded as a treatment for the 'hardware' components if the brain is viewed as a computer. Psychiatry handles the 'software,' and neurology is in between, dealing with both.

I truly found my calling during the second six months of 1996 when I worked as a service registrar in neurology. I could be called by the emergency department or doctors from outside the hospital from anywhere in the state, at any time, every second day and night. Virtually every call-night involved returning to the hospital to see new patients and administer the necessary care. This added up to thousands of hours spent in the hospital. This kind of medical workload is now outlawed in most countries, and there is no doubt it was highly dangerous for patients as well as the doctors sentenced to this on-call nightmare. Kirsten remembers how I would flinch at the sound of a telephone ringing, with the expectation that yet another trip back to the hospital would be required. The saving grace was the enormous experience I gained.

## Neurology training

In that era, neurology training, like many other specialty programs in Australia, was really an apprenticeship. There were two core years of training, rotating around the main local teaching hospitals, and then an elective year, which could be pretty much anything although a stint overseas was the preferred option. This didn't stop us going ahead and starting our family. James was born in October 1997 and Matthew in March 1999. Numerous generations of Australian neurology trainees have travelled to the UK, USA, and more recently Canada, to undertake fellowships to broaden experience and put the finishing touches on their training. My path took me to the Mayo Clinic in Rochester, Minnesota.

## USA here we come

The Blacker family arrived in Rochester, Minnesota in mid-June 2001. We had arranged to take over a rental house less than a mile from St Mary's Hospital from the preceding Australian fellow, a Queenslander. There is a long tradition of Australians doing a one-year fellowship at the Mayo Clinic in Rochester, so the program is very well organised, and the opportunities for research and academic papers were incredible; I published 13 papers as a result of my time at Mayo and gladly committed to a second year in order to undertake a stroke fellowship. There were offers for me to stay longer, but a position was coming up in Perth for me, and we were all ready to go home. Despite having many friends and colleagues in the USA, I didn't want to live there long term, and I didn't want our kids to grow up there.

## Back to Australia

I commenced full-time practice at Sir Charles Gairdner Hospital in August 2003. That was the same month the Therapeutic Goods Administration approved tissue plasminogen activator (tPA) for use in stroke. This is the 'clot busting' drug that dramatically changed stroke treatment forever. This was great timing, since I'd had a solid grounding in using tPA while at Mayo. I dived straight into setting up an acute stroke team, establishing a local protocol and starting to use it routinely. (See chapter *Hanging on for one more year*.)

## Losing the Minnesota lard

With all this activity I was aware that I had been neglecting my own physical fitness and health, and had been doing this for almost ten years. I'd always been very active and played a lot of sports. My golf game peaked in about the third year of university, and I was still playing competitions and pennants until my intern year. I had a swimming teaching certificate and taught vacation swimming classes in my first two summer breaks at university. I even competed in the swim legs of some team triathlons. All this disappeared with a decade of study and work.

When I returned from the US, I weighed more than 90 kilograms. The cold Minnesota weather, the large American servings and some home sickness comfort eating all contributed. It struck me that I was now sitting in a clinic encouraging stroke patients to live a healthy lifestyle, and I wasn't doing that myself. It was time for me to make some changes.

The simple thing to do was to start walking. I lived near Lake Gwelup, in the northern Perth suburbs, and there were several different tracks around it with loops between 2.5 to 3.5 kilometres. Somewhere along the way, the walking accelerated into a little jog which soon became an entire 3.5-kilometre circuit. I bought a runners' watch and kept track of my times and distances and started to keep records on an Excel sheet. I'd settle into a steady pace, initially aiming to complete one kilometre in six minutes, and eventually chipping this down to five minutes. I was very pleased when I completed one half marathon averaging less than five minutes per kilometre. Running made me feel alive and healthy, and obliterated the 'Minnesota lard.' After about a year of running, I started to participate in some events, and joined the Perth Marathon Club. This didn't mean you had to run a marathon; there were numerous events from 5 kilometres to the marathon distance, but the marathon became my goal. I studied training regimens recommended in running magazines and was pleased to learn the recommended training distances were well within what I was doing already. I became obsessed about doing my 'Ks' and at one stage I was averaging 80–100 kilometres per week. Over about a four-year span I completed six full marathons, including one on my fortieth birthday and dozens of half marathons, including a stint where for about twenty consecutive weekends I ran a half marathon distance training run each Sunday morning. I did this very early, returning home just as the rest of my family was getting up, so I didn't miss out on any activities. I could even be on call for the hospital by keeping to routes close to home in case I had to dash back and go into work. However, I was not vigilant with stretching or resting, and initially I attributed an emerging problem with my right foot to those factors.

## My funky right foot

During the last 10 kilometres of my second marathon I felt a peculiar twisting and tightening of my right leg, especially the foot. It wasn't overtly painful, but it was unpleasant, and made it difficult to run. Initially I wasn't over-concerned, until it started to occur consistently at shorter times and distances. It would also happen if I was pushing the pace. Sometimes I could speed up and finish a race before it struck, but that was a juggling act. If I really concentrated on my form and posture, and ran steadily, I could stave if off, but once it happened, a full-blown attack would force me to slow considerably. If I ran sideways, or even backwards for a while, I could delay it. Sometimes I would stop and try some stretching. I obtained a hip x-ray and consulted a podiatrist and a physiotherapist; neither had any answers. Observers thought I had a cramp, and I went along with that, rather than the tricky diagnosis of exercise induced dystonia. With the passage of time, it even started to impact brisk paced walking, especially if I did this when I was tired, or in the afternoons. I sought other ways to maintain fitness in addition to walking, such as swimming, and later on light weights and yoga. Fortunately, I had achieved my goal of getting to a healthy weight and building an above average level of cardiovascular fitness. The next thing was to maintain it.

This form of dystonia can sometimes precede PD[2], but I had no other symptoms. It was very difficult to find any useful information in the medical literature to indicate what the chances of developing PD might be in this situation. Even though I have a tendency to fear the worst, especially in my patients, it wasn't something I was concerned about. It is well recognised that medical practitioners are apt to worry themselves about the possibility of illnesses and I was perhaps conscious of appearing neurotic. Whatever the reason, at this stage I didn't think there was anything I should consult with my neurological colleagues about.

## Early experience with Parkinson's disease

I'll back track a little now to describe what I knew about PD before I began to develop the classic symptoms that ultimately made the diagnosis clear. I obviously knew about PD as a medical student and junior doctor. One early memory was during a rural elective in between my fifth and sixth years of medical school where I worked for about six weeks with an experienced general surgeon. I recall seeing an elderly man in the surgical clinic and noted features that seemed to me to suggest Parkinson's disease. After the surgical issues had been dealt with, and the patient left the room, I asked the surgeon about PD, and was a little shocked that he hadn't noticed, and was reluctant to take the issue up.

In my second year after graduation, I did a general medical rotation at Perth's Hollywood Hospital, which at that time was a veterans' hospital. The unit I was working on was run by a neurologist, who also covered the general medicine service. There was an outpatient neurology clinic, where there was a large number of elderly patients with PD. I found it depressing to see these proud Diggers, who had once fought for their country, to be so debilitated, shuffling slowly in to be examined. I was also frustrated to see that apart from a sympathetic ear, and a few tweaks of the medication, it didn't seem like a lot was being done for them.

During the early to mid-1990s, Sir Charles Gairdner Hospital began offering neurosurgical interventions for movement disorders, ultimately building a strong and well regarded deep brain stimulation (DBS) program for PD. This is the operation where a thin electrical wire is carefully inserted into strategic small structures deep within the brain, some as small as less than 3 millimetres. An electrical current passes through these wires, adjusted in order to damp down some of the excessive brain activity characteristically seen in PD, but also in other disorders. During my rotations, I had the opportunity to see some of this. One striking memory I have, is seeing a patient with a severe, incapacitating essential tremor who was struggling to use utensils to eat. I had a role in working through the settings adjusting his stimulator shortly after it was inserted. Watching his violent tremor coming to stillness when the optimal setting was found was spectacular, and inspiring.

As described earlier, I had gained a lot of experience with acute hospital neurology, but the exposure to PD and other movement disorders in the outpatients clinic was not so prominent. There was a new comprehensive movement disorders clinic next door to the hospital, at the Australian Neuromuscular Institute, later known as the

West Australian Neuroscience Research Institute, where I became the medical director in 2014, and then again renamed the Perron Institute. Trainees were always welcome to attend these clinics to gain experience, but with the punishing inpatient service workload and arduous on-call, it was very difficult to escape the pressure of the hospital to attend these clinics, where a goldmine of clinical experience was available.

This meant that when I saw a PwP, it was usually in the acute inpatient setting, when something terrible had gone wrong, such as a delirium or psychosis, often triggered by some other intervening medical issue. I vividly recall a psychotic PD patient smashing a window on the ward with a chair; a window with thick glass that no-one thought could possibly be broken. The result was that at this stage in my career I had a very skewed view of PD, and never felt comfortable with the diagnosis or management. There was scant opportunity to see a lot of PD patients in the general neurology outpatient setting, or follow them for any great length of time. Little did I know how this would one day change dramatically. Compounding my lack of confidence about PD was the fact the movement disorder specialists I had interaction with, all seemed to be of daunting intellect and great neurological prowess. They seemed to be regarded as the premier subspecialists, with special knowledge of the rare and complex. I thought that I didn't have the knowledge, expertise or the patience to be a PD expert and regarded myself more as a 'tradesman' neurologist, familiar with the common conditions in large volumes. Besides, I really had the stroke bug and had a plan to 'save the world from stroke'; a catchphrase Kirsten and I came up with as I departed once again towards the emergency department. This was a big job, and I was engrossed in it, and remain heavily involved in the field, although from about 2019 onward I have progressively pulled back, as I will describe later.

## More symptoms emerge

For several years, my only issue was the exercise induced foot dystonia. Sometime in early 2016 I started to note a tremor of my right hand and right foot, initially only when very anxious or stressed. More than likely my ongoing high intake of caffeine was a contributing factor, and for quite a while I hoped that was all it was. There were some episodes when shaking did become obvious. For example, on a flight to a family holiday a passenger seated in the back row passed out while vomiting. Kirsten and I provided some assistance. Even though I have answered the in-flight call 'is there a doctor on board?' at least half a dozen times, it is always a bit stressful and nerve wracking. After the situation came under control, I noticed my right hand visibly shaking. On another flight to an overseas conference, Kirsten and I again teamed up with several other medical professionals to assist a person who was having a seizure. I was perhaps less nervous dealing with an emergency within my own field, but again with a surge of adrenaline my right hand began to shake. It wasn't long, to my great annoyance, that I started to notice the same problem when playing golf.

## Impact on golf

As described earlier, I've been playing golf since childhood. I live less than a kilometre from Lake Karrinyup Country Club, one of Australia's best golf courses, where I have been a member since 2005. When my boys finished high school, and my career was more established, I started to play again regularly, after a decade or so of infrequent play. I went from playing one or two games per month to one or two per week, and some of the form of my youth returned; I gradually got my handicap down to 6 again. Golf is not an easy game, and as my PD symptoms started to emerge, it started to get more and more difficult. I was able to minimise the impact of tremor by altering my putting technique; swapping to a left hand under grip, so that any shaking wouldn't really impact on the stroke – I'm not sure what I will do if both become involved. Perhaps the biggest problem though, was the slowness at moving my right hand and leg. Balance was also an issue; one day I was lining up on the practice range, took a few steps backwards and managed to tumble over, spraining my outstretched wrist. It hurt for several months. The most embarrassing problems at golf were very simple. Just placing the ball on the tee was difficult, sometimes taking several attempts. Another issue was marking the ball on the green. For non-golfing readers, when golfers are on the putting green, and their ball is in the way of other players, you place a small plastic marker or coin on the ground to mark the position of the ball before picking it up to get it out of the way. My usual practice was to use a five cent piece as a marker, with my coins being in my right pocket (and my tees in my left pocket). I had incredible trouble reaching into my right pocket to find the coins and my hand would 'stick' in my pocket. The other issue was that troublesome right foot and leg, which would start playing its dystonic tricks towards the end of the round, especially when walking up the steep hills that finish each of the nine holes at Karrinyup. All these little things sound trivial, but were examples of PD and its core features. Little wonder my handicap steadily blew out from 6 to 12; my proud run of being in single figures for over thirty-five years was over.

## Symptoms at work

While the impact on my golf was annoying, when it started to influence my work, I began to realise that I would have to do something about it soon. My previously energetic bounding gait which would include zooming up several flights of stairs as the team trailed behind, was becoming an ungainly trudge across the hospital. When colleagues commented, I'd brush it off, saying I was a bit sore from running too much. I developed a habit of holding my small exam bag (proudly brought back from the Mayo Clinic – a symbol amongst neurologists of doing time there) in the crook of my bent and slow moving right elbow. My handwriting, never good to begin with, was becoming a laborious scrawl. Initially, I minimised the issue by laughing it off as 'typical doctors handwriting,' and by making a conscious effort to be more concise. I would try to complete as many forms as I could before the patients came into my office. Looking back through my outpatient notes, I could clearly see the deterioration. At times, I started using my left hand to move the right hand with the pen. What became more disturbing was my observation that many of my PD patients were moving more freely than I was. One thing that neurologists do as part of the routine examination is to demonstrate rapid alternating tapping movements of the fingers. This can reveal a lot of information about the integrity of the motor pathways and what is known as the extra-pyramidal system, which is impacted in PD. It was apparent that my non-dominant left hand was quicker, and more dexterous, than my right.

There were some non-motor issues as well. I was finding the stress of work difficult to deal with, and found my mood to be fluctuating, with a tendency towards grumpiness. Some of my long-standing patients could see that something was wrong, and I was impressed how one of my patients (not a PD patient) made the diagnosis when some of my colleagues hadn't even suspected it.

## Time to start treatment

Having described all these symptoms in detail, readers might ask why I took so long to seek an independent consultation and commence treatment. It was more than two years after the slowness and stiffness became problematic that I sought help. In some public health systems (including Australia's), people with similar symptoms can wait this long for a specialist appointment. I have a whole host of reasons for the delay, which all sound like weak excuses now. The first was that it had all started so slowly and insidiously. I had hoped that the exercise induced dystonia would remain just that, and symptoms of PD would not emerge. The tremor was only intermittent and short lived, and not a consistent problem. I also had the fear that I was being a paranoid hypochondriac and was imagining symptoms. I didn't want to put Kirsten and the boys through the stress that I knew a formal diagnosis would bring, unless it was a certainty. A big factor of course was my career. At first, I was confident I was still managing, and in no danger of harming patients. Thankfully, not being a surgeon or a proceduralist, my work was almost entirely cognitive and I had found ways to compensate for the deficiencies. The handwriting issue was becoming a problem, and becoming more and more energy sapping. I gradually came to be certain that I wasn't imagining things and this was really looking like PD. This made me feel guilty that I was deceiving people when they noticed a change in me, and I denied there was anything wrong.

There was also the debate about when to commence treatment with medications, with concerns that early commencement with drugs, particularly L-dopa, could lead to the earlier appearance of medication complications. Over the last few years these concerns have been dispelled, and many movement disorder specialists are now advocating earlier treatment, particularly to optimise the PD patient's ability to participate in exercise – the one thing that seems to slow progression. In retrospect, I wish I had commenced symptomatic treatment with L-dopa earlier; I regret missing out on the benefits it has provided. So finally, my increasing symptoms, which were interfering with several aspects of my life, drove me to overcome the procrastination and seek help by getting a formal diagnosis and starting treatment.

I thought I should start with an MRI of the brain. While this is not necessary for the diagnosis of PD in classic cases, I felt I should do this, and then get on and see a neurologist colleague. I'd had MRIs before, once when I was a control subject in some work on developing functional MRI protocols. (I went on to co-author a paper[3] where we worked with speech pathologists to develop a protocol for localising the language areas of the brain and later did a small study of stroke patients with dysphasia [impaired language]). So, I was familiar with being inside the MRI tunnel. This one seemed to be a bit different; again, there was anxiety, and the right sided tremor appeared. The MRI staff were fantastic and the neuroradiologist called me the next day, reassuring me the scan was entirely normal. He said, 'It looks like you've been looking after your brain.' I recall staring at my MRI, and feeling strangely frustrated that it looked so normal, but clearly wasn't working properly. I had heard patients talk about this frustration, and had been unable to understand it; I thought they should be grateful to have normal anatomy. But now, confronted with a clear scan, I too felt this paradoxical disappointment at having no visual evidence to explain my symptoms.

The next task was to choose a colleague to see. Perth neurologists are a very small group, and there are a limited number of movement disorder subspecialists. Given that I didn't think there was any diagnostic difficulty, my choice was based around some other complex factors. I wanted someone a little separate from my day-to-day work, someone I respected, and I also didn't want to stress out one of my previous trainees by asking them to look after me. I wrote a referral letter, briefly outlining many of the symptoms I have previously described here. I made an appointment, as the last patient, late on a Friday afternoon. Kirsten and I went in together. I was surprised at how nervous I was, and again the right sided tremor was there for us all to see. I could feel the rigidity as he carefully examined my limbs, and my slowed finger-tapping on the right all made the clinical diagnosis straightforward.

The diagnosis should not have been a surprise, but it still hit me hard, and there were some tears. On the positive side, he gave me a script for Madopar, which I was happy to try. He was independently of the opinion we should go straight to L-dopa. I was not keen to start with a dopamine agonist such as pramipexole; I have seen patients get sleepy on this, and suffer impulse control disorders. I already have obsessive tendencies and don't enjoy any feeling of sedation, so am probably not a good candidate for these medications.

I vividly recall taking my first dose of Madopar one afternoon, and testing my right-hand finger tapping. After about forty-five minutes I could feel a clear difference, with the movements becoming smoother and quicker. A few further doses confirmed that I was indeed responding to the medication. I was pleasantly surprised by this. For some reason my expectations were low. I had waited so long to start, it seemed almost too good to be true. Even though I had seen good responses in patients before, I have also seen patients with little improvement, so I felt very lucky to be obtaining benefit. My walking also improved, and in the days and weeks to follow, I enjoyed a new sense of freedom of movement.

The only downside was nausea. It took me a few weeks to get into a regular routine of taking it three times a day, and it took about that long for the nausea to settle. Nausea is such a horrible feeling. When you are dealing with the emotional stress of a new diagnosis, and starting a new treatment, nausea is the last thing you need. Oral L-dopa crosses into the brain and then is metabolised to dopamine. L-dopa is usually combined with another agent, either benserazide (in the brand Maopar) or carbidopa (in Sinemet and Kinson). They are the second part of the dose written on the medication labelling. For example, the 25 milligrams in Madopar 100/25. These components inhibit the breakdown of L-dopa into dopamine in the blood outside the brain. This allows more L-dopa to reach the brain, and reduces nausea that results from L-dopa being metabolised into dopamine outside the brain. Probably 75–100 milligrams of benserazide or carbidopa is required to counter the nausea, so when starting off at a low dose, such as one 100/25 milligram tablet three times a day, there is only just enough of this. Reassurance that the nausea will abate is important.

It took me a while to get the rhythm of the medication regimen going. Just like any patient, I had a bit of trouble remembering doses, and had the frustration of thinking 'have I taken it or not?' In that situation I might take half a tablet, so I wouldn't be too far off the mark either way. I had never thought of recommending that until I had to take them myself! Another strategy was to carry a day's supply with me, so I could avoid the uncertainty. Pretty soon I started carrying the number I needed, plus an extra, in case I dropped or lost one. I arranged a supply of tablets all over the place, including a bottle in the kitchen, my car and one at work. I have numerous small plastic containers that were initially for ear plugs, each filled with about eight capsules. On weekends or when going out I usually have one in my pocket. At work and at golf I have so much other stuff in my pockets there is not enough room, so I keep a supply in my small black neuro exam bag from the Mayo clinic (one of my precious possessions), and my golf bag; my favourite bag. I am paranoid about running out, because the feeling of being 'off' is terrible, so I am fastidious about keeping my scripts up to date. I prefer the Madopar capsules because they are easier to swallow than the tablets. The advantage of the tablets is that they can be broken into smaller pieces in order to make dose adjustments, whereas capsules cannot. When I travel I usually pack an extra bottle of tablets. I do this in case I lose my main supply while in a location where I couldn't easily obtain a script, having tablets that I could break apart and 'ration' the supply out.

I doubt I would have ever imagined these nuances if I wasn't taking this medication myself.

## Reaction to the diagnosis

The weeks following the formal diagnosis and commencement of medication were difficult. Even though I knew it was coming, to hear it being confirmed still had a powerful effect. On the positive side, it confirmed that I was not imagining the symptoms, and it wasn't something else – a few irrational thoughts about alternative, more sinister pathologies had been swirling around in the back of my mind. There was also some validation of my own diagnosis; not that there was much doubt when the symptoms and signs were assessed objectively, but I had started to doubt myself. What I found particularly difficult was a shift in my thinking about the future. My previous mental picture was of looking forward to a very active retirement, perhaps still doing some private work and research, but also enjoying a lot of travel with Kirsten. In addition, I'd hoped to finally have some time to put in extra practice and improve my golf game, and even get good enough to play in some amateur tournaments again and perhaps in senior pennants. I suddenly felt that all of this wasn't going to happen, and that because of the nature of PD, I would inevitably progress and get functionally worse because that is what is supposed to happen in PD. This feeling of the future I had planned being taken away, was probably the worst part of the early post diagnosis time.

What I had failed to realise, was how much function I had already lost, and that with medication and improvement in my fitness and strength, I could get a lot of that back, and return to a higher level of functioning than where I had been at the time of diagnosis. I think I reached this point sometime during 2021.

# 'Coming out' – revealing the diagnosis

Kirsten and my sons were incredibly supportive. We tried to be as positive as possible, especially for the sake of our boys. Kirsten was always there to help me through the times where things got a bit tough. Early on I advised other close family members and friends directly. There were mixed reactions, with some people becoming very upset and concerned. I felt bad about distressing these people, and found that quite draining. I came to learn that quite often I would not be in the mood to 'reveal' because it did require quite an emotional effort. I sent a detailed e-mail to my work colleagues to get it all done in one hit. I was surprised that it came as a shock to most of them. Even the neurologist that I consulted said he hadn't noted anything when seeing me every few weeks at inter-hospital meetings. I hadn't realised how much energy I was consuming in concealing my symptoms. Previously, when people had asked about my gait issues, I came up with some excuse about muscular soreness from exercise. Now, if it was appropriate and someone asked, I just told them. I was uncomfortable giving misleading answers, and I also didn't want people to think that a neurologist had missed making an obvious diagnosis in himself. To some degree, finally revealing what was going on was liberating.

It did come at a difficult time at work, though. One of my colleagues suddenly resigned as the Head of Department of Neurology. He had been worn down by a very stressful job in an environment with limited staff resources and little support from medical administration, as well as chronic under-recognition of some of the world class clinical work and research that was going on. I had been acting Head of Department on numerous occasions over many years, and was seen as the next in line. I had tried to indicate that I didn't want the position, and had already started to reduce my public hospital commitments, focusing more on research at the Perron Institute and private practice. Such was the level of crisis at the hospital, that there was a very real threat to the functioning of the department. Part of my motivation for a blanket disclosure to all of my colleagues was to explain to them my reluctance to take over as the head. I had hoped that someone else would take on the role. This didn't occur, and I felt that I would probably be more stressed if I did not take on this task, as I didn't want to see the work I had been doing for many years disintegrate. So, I took the role on, with the clearly stated proviso that I would only do this for a year and would almost immediately start mentoring a successor. I continued in the role through to January 2020, and helped to stabilise the situation, bringing in a number of logistical changes to the way the service was run. I am satisfied with what I accomplished – but hated every minute of the role. I was there purely because of my knowledge of the hospital system, rather than any desire to be a leader. I had clear ideas about some big-picture changes that would benefit patients and staff alike, and I was happy to develop and institute these. The logistics of rosters, leave requests, signing off on paysheets, meeting with medical administration and dealing with complaints, while all very important, were things I really didn't want to do. They were far removed from patient care and research; my main interests in medicine. At the same time, because of the restructure, I was one of the three neurologists in the department purely covering the acute stroke service which, during that time, became one of the highest volume stroke services in Australia.

My already fragmented, light sleep became much worse. My insomnia had several precipitants. There were my ruminations over the future, with questions about how quickly the PD would progress; if I would be able to work and what would my quality of life be like? How would it impact on Kirsten and the boys? There were also work worries. I had a jigsaw puzzle of juggling staff FTE (full time equivalents) allocations in my head at all times. My vivid dreams escalated, and I noted that taking long acting Madopar to combat decreased nocturnal mobility seemed to worsen the dreams; there was a lot of yelling. Unlike Sigmund Freud, I didn't have any problems waking up to interpret dreams; in fact, quite often the dreams woke me, scared, and with a pounding heart that would make it very difficult to get back to sleep. Kirsten had her own insomnia issues with menopausal flushing and heat intolerance. In addition, I was still doing on-call at least once a week, with the inevitable after midnight calls, all serving to deepen our sleep disruption. For a while, this disruption distressed me, especially when it impacted on the next day with fatigue. Gradually, I simply came to accept the situation, and if I needed a short nap the following day, I'd just sneak off to do this. Sometimes, I found a quiet back room in the clinic somewhere to nap, but that was not very relaxing. A better option was a nap in my car, so I would park in a distant corner of the hospital multi-storey car park, where I could quietly take a nap to recharge, and then return for several hours more work and finish the day. Usually, I slept for just five to 7 minutes, with a disproportionate improvement in energy levels.

Unfortunately, such sleep disruptions can lead to a migraine the following day. I've had migraines since childhood. I have a very distinct memory of my mother taking me to a general practitioner when I was about eleven years of age with a severe headache, vomiting, and numbness down the left side of my body. In my mid to late teens, I came to recognise a tell-tale aura of shimmering lights flashing through my vision, invariably to be followed later by nausea and a pounding head. Every now and then I would have to call Kirsten and ask her to pick me up from work because I could not drive in such a state. I've had numerous rounds of golf destroyed by migraine auras. Often, I'd recognise them and quickly take aspirin and caffeine, which would modify the pain, but not the visual disturbance. (It's very difficult to hit the ball when you can't actually see it!) The disrupted sleep meant that a migraine always seemed to be on the cards.

## Hanging on for one tough year

The year 2019 was a tough one. Not only was I adjusting to having PD, but the work volume and stress levels were higher than ever. I kept up my exercise, walking a minimum of 15 kilometres per week, using a smart phone app to keep a record. I wasn't pushing myself, I was just keeping up that distance, and not feeling particularly fit. I was still trying to play golf once or twice a week, and was pleased the Madopar was making a difference; I was able to walk more easily and swing a little faster. My golf handicap was coming down again, settling back to 7 or 8, and I was happy to be playing a bit better and enjoying it. I found myself using golf as a way of trying to forget about all the stress, at least for a few hours. One of my former trainees, who is now a movement disorder neurologist, monitors his golfing patients' handicaps as a marker of how their PD is progressing; I think that is a great idea. Several years previously, I had started taking Wednesday mornings off to play golf. I'd tee off with a regular group just after dawn, then shower, change, dose up with caffeine and rush to get to the midday stroke meeting where we reviewed most of the stroke cases of the preceding week. I'd then rush to clinic, and then back home in time for yoga.

Kirsten and I had a small foray into yoga while the kids were still at school, but didn't keep it up. With both boys out of home from 2016, we started to do yoga again regularly, and I started to find it beneficial for my physical health and mental state. Numerous elements of yoga appeared to be useful, including the meditative aspects and breathing, as well as the balance work and focus on developing core muscle strength. I find the best feature for me comes from the prolonged, deep stretching practiced in yin yoga. I try to do at least one session of yin per week, and find that my rigidity, which can be quite painful at times, will worsen if I don't.

Around the same time as I started taking Wednesday mornings off, Kirsten wisely instituted a Wednesday date night rule; banning me from touching my laptop, making calls or doing work chores on Wednesday night. This strategy preserved me, and I found myself working efficiently on Tuesday afternoons and nights, knowing I would get a break on Wednesday.

Even though acute stroke is my subspecialty and I had a major role in establishing the service, I was finding the work increasingly stressful. One issue was the relentless and growing workload. In 2019 there were more than 1,000 acute stroke calls at Sir Charles Gairdner Hospital. Stroke is an urgent condition; decisions have to be made immediately, often with incomplete and changing information while sleep deprived. Many of the decisions are true life-and-death decisions. Often, the stroke pager would go off again, as I was walking to the hospital car park to leave at the end of a long day. This felt particularly tough late on a Tuesday afternoon if I had just started to get a glimpse of my treasured Wednesday. I'd turn back towards the emergency department, pausing at the vending machine to buy yet another Diet Coke to gulp down as I walked to the CT scan room to meet the team and make the decisions. My caffeine consumption was enormous; I felt like I was a slave to the coffee bean, experiencing mood swings, withdrawal headaches and insomnia. The on-call roster (and nature of my work being mainly focused on acute stroke) had me constantly feeling tightly wound up. The weekends of on-call were becoming a torture. I felt like I couldn't even go to the toilet without the phone ringing. The emotional drain of seeing many people with severe life-changing illnesses, and the suffering of their loved ones, was energy sapping. I was burnt out before I'd even heard of the term. I was also aware of how moody and grumpy I could get when on call. I particularly disliked the fact that when I was doing a weekend on call, I was soon thinking about how many hours were left until it was over.

Kirsten's Wednesday plan helped me survive 2019, although towards the end I stopped getting up before dawn to play golf because I was simply too tired. The other psychological ploy I used was constant forward planning; knowing I had a successor for the head of department position, Thankfully, my plans worked out, and from early 2020 I was able to back off my public hospital commitment with a corresponding reduction in stress levels. From June 2020, I reduced to just one full day a week as well as some on-call, and I started taking Wednesdays off completely. The remainder of my professional time was split between private practice and the Perron Institute. This also allowed for a large increase in the time I was able to spend working on my physical fitness, which I will describe in more detail a little later.

# Coming out 'big'

In mid-2020, I took the 'coming out' to another level. One of the many journals I read regularly, *Practical Neurology*, from the *British Medical Journal* group, has a section, 'My neurological illness,' which publishes essays about physicians with neurological conditions. I looked through previous issues and couldn't find an article on PD, so it seemed like a logical place for me to submit an article[4]. I found it quite cathartic, although the limit of 800 words ensured it was succinct. It was one of the easiest things I have ever written, since I knew the subject (me) fairly thoroughly. The response from the editors was very complimentary, and it was published quite quickly, with only a few subtle revisions required. It was published on-line in the middle on 2020, and the response was rapid, and more emotive than I could possibly have imagined. I received dozens of beautiful and heartfelt e-mails from colleagues all around the world, including former trainees and colleagues in the USA and Europe.

A second flurry of responses followed the distribution of the hard copy of the journal in October. Several other physicians with PD sent messages and we exchanged experiences; one colleague with PD from Ireland even had some recommendations for a brand of golf clubs. There were colleagues who stated they felt relieved to learn that someone else was going through similar issues. Some were effusive about the article, calling it brave and courageous, which was nice of them, but seemed strange to me. I was simply telling my experience as it is; I couldn't see any obvious bravery or potential downside to open disclosure. Maybe there was a risk that patients and colleagues might no longer trust or listen to me because I had PD. I have concerns in the longer term regarding the potential for cognitive decline, but I trusted my treating neurologist to keep this under objective review. I've found the experience almost liberating, and it has helped me to focus on what I want to achieve in the final years of my career. I feel that I have a responsibility to the PD community to make the most of my unique situation to assist in improving care and research into the condition.

This feeling was at the forefront of my mind when I was invited to contribute to the World Federation of Neurology (WFN), World Brain Day, on 22 July 2020, the theme being PD. I recorded a short video outlining my view on the impact of PD from a patient perspective. I was honoured when the president of the WFN, and my main mentor during training, Bill Carroll introduced the webinar and showed my video as the first message after his introduction.

In the same week, Channel 7 Perth ran a television news story for World Brain Day, featuring the non-contact boxing exercise program I developed as a PD treatment, and which I will be describing in detail in the second section of this book. The interest generated by this story quickly provided us with a large number of PwP eager to be involved in research; which was precisely what we were hoping for. The story was also shown on the national news bulletins. I thought I couldn't 'come out' any more than this – but as it turned out, I could. A couple of months later, the public relations staff at the Perron Institute approached me, wanting to know if I would help with a television advertisement as part of a media campaign to bolster the profile of the institute. The ultimate objective of this was to enhance fundraising and donations, which would be fed back into the non-profit organisation's research budget. I have always been acutely aware of the difficult task most scientists in Australia have to maintain funding for research, so I had no hesitation in agreeing to help. The message of the advertisement was that in middle age, a range of neurological conditions – such as PD, Alzheimer's and stroke – loom, and that the research and clinical trials at the Perron Institute are looking at practical ways to help patients with these conditions. The advertising producer wanted a middle-aged person to portray a patient with a neurological condition. I figured there was no need to pay an actor when I was the exact profile they wanted, grey and thinning hair included.

There were a couple of short planning sessions and a few e-mails which all seemed straightforward. However, I had not anticipated how intense the day of filming would be. The location was to be on one of Perth's local beaches, City Beach. Poor weather resulted in the first planned date being cancelled. The second date proved to be perfect, with initially sunny weather conditions, later followed by dark clouds gathering on the horizon at sunset, which was ideal for the theme of the ad. I decided to skip my afternoon dose of Madopar, with a view to making the tremor and gait disturbance more authentic. (I recall reading that Michael J Fox was criticised for adjusting his doses before appearing at a US Senate enquiry in order to make his symptoms more apparent. My symptoms were more subtle than Michael's, but certainly had an impact.) I am not really a beachgoer, and I suddenly realised that I hadn't walked on sand since my PD symptoms had become prominent. Walking on soft beach sand is quite a challenge in the off-state, so the gait disturbance seen in the final ad is definitely genuine; no acting required. The filming was interesting, but exhausting, and gave me a tremendous appreciation and respect for the television production process. Over the next few months, the advertisement was featured during prime time, with the local channels providing a generously discounted rate. The following year, during the Tokyo Olympics, it seemed to be playing most nights. I found it a bit of a shock to see my own face on television. Plenty of my patients saw it and recognised me, even though the filming was done without me wearing my trademark glasses. While it achieved the goal of promoting the Perron Institute, there was a downside; a couple of my patients were upset at seeing me like this, not having realised I had PD. I don't regret doing it, but I was happy when it faded from public memory and I stopped getting asked, 'are you in that TV ad?'

# FIGHTing PD

# Taking up the FIGHT against PD

At the start of 2020, before COVID, I could feel relief and rejuvenation. In January I handed over the Head of Department responsibilities, and soon had some improvement in my insomnia. I finally felt like I had some time to devote to learning more about PD and focusing on my own health. During 2019, I had saved dozens of articles on PD, putting them aside for a time when I had a chance to absorb them. I started listening to webinars and podcasts on PD on the way to work. If I had an hour of insomnia I'd read more or watch YouTube clips on PD topics. I found plenty of interesting materials from the MJ Fox and Davis Phinney Foundations, as well as in medical journals I already subscribed to. I was particularly interested in the literature on PD and exercise, and began to study anything I could find on that topic. I was especially interested in the work done by Jay Alberts from Cleveland and Bastiaan Bloem from the Netherlands, and I read many of their papers and watched their lectures and presentations. Jay's work on cycling and forced exercise[5] fascinated me, and Bastiaan's devotion to the overall care of PD patients is incredible. I became convinced that physical exercise was a key component of PD treatment, and in many ways perhaps the most important element. Not only does it have the best data for any disease modulating effect, it provides a definite sense of empowerment for PwP, rewarding them by making them feel better and motivating them to take on the fight themselves. From my reading I realised that I wasn't doing enough exercise, but just treading water to maintain a constant level.

I was also enjoying being able to devote more attention to my role as Medical Director of the Perron Institute. The enthusiasm and curiosity of neuroscientists and researchers energised me. This was a great counterbalance to the frazzled stress of public hospital work. Now the opportunity to focus more intently without the stroke pager going off in the middle of a consultation, allowed me to enjoy private practice more. I am certain that divesting some of my workload and reducing stress was highly beneficial for me.

## Rai Fazio – a boxer joins the fight

Shortly before the COVID calamity began to impact everything in March, an alignment of circumstances and opportunities (some people call it fate), occurred that would shape my future, redirect my career and significantly improve my health.

The story of how Rai and I were drawn together is remarkable and full of co-incidences. Some have described us as 'the professor and the pugilist.' Rai probably never imagined that he would be reading scientific articles and contributing to academic meetings and papers; and I never imagined I would be looking at video clips of Mike Tyson.

As you have read, I have always been interested and enthused about sports. As well as my ongoing addiction to golf, and era of long-distance running, I'm one of those Australians meeting the description of a cricket tragic, and played a bit of club cricket to a reasonable level. I also played a bit of casual tennis and always enjoyed it. Although not an enthusiastic beachgoer, I gained a swimming instructors' qualification which I used as a summer job in my first few years of medical school to earn a bit of money; mainly to finance golf. Boxing was not on the list of sports I was interested in. I did admire the athleticism and fitness, but I think the head trauma and brutality turned me off it, so I had no understanding of the tactics and strategy. In my burst of reading about exercise and PD, I had read about boxing, and particularly the Rock Steady program popular in North America. I watched a few videos and was struck by how much enjoyment the PwP seemed to have, engaging in large, enthusiastic group sessions.

Rai Fazio was born to be a boxer. His father, Joe, was a successful amateur boxer in Italy and a member of the national boxing squad for the 1960 Rome Olympics, although unfortunately, he did not get to compete. Upon emigrating to Australia in the early 1960s he opened the

Balga Boxing Club in Perth's northern suburbs. He trained boxers there until his death in 2022.

Rai recalls starting to box from the age of four and had his first fight in 1972. Part of the training regimen was a detailed warm-up that Joe had learnt from an Italian boxing coach many years before. It consisted of methodical loosening of joints and muscles from head to toe, and included various balancing, movement and aerobic components. It's a much more detailed and vigorous preparation than the rudimentary exercises done at many boxing facilities prior to sparring or getting into the ring. A few years after we started, Rai noted that some parts looked very much like moves made in Thai Chi, only done much more rapidly. Thai Chi has been shown to be effective for PD, and there is a paper[6] on this in the prestigious *New England Journal of Medicine*. Rai learnt early that movement, balance and full utilisation of the ring are just as important as throwing punches.

Very soon, Rai was competing, and winning against much older and larger opponents. He quickly picked up several golden gloves state and national boxing titles. Rai and I laughed when he told me how in 1983, at the age of sixteen, he won an Australian national boxing title; the same year I won the State Junior High School Mathematics Competition! What a contrast! However, it was not as nerdy as it sounds as it was for a project on the mathematics in sport.

Rai had the skills, talent and knowledge to go a long way in boxing, but he was worried about how the sport could affect his health. After one famous victory, his friends were asking him about some details of the fight that he was shocked he couldn't remember. This made him decide to get out. As might be expected, this was not a popular decision with his father. The angst of this and Rai's story was the subject of a 2008 movie, *Two Fists One Heart,* written by Rai himself. One of the stars was Tim Minchin, one of Kirsten's favourite Australian actors and performers. Rai described to me how he came to write the movie, and the connections he made with some big names in Hollywood. The story behind writing the movie could almost become a movie in itself. Rai had an acting role in the movie, and later had small parts in some Australian television series, including *Underbelly.*

The movie, and acting, couldn't pay the bills, so he got back to what he knew: boxing. This time it was as a coach and trainer. His knowledge of the sport, and a wonderful ability to teach it with his great communication skills, made him a natural trainer. He soon recognised problems with some of the basic boxing training equipment such as punching bags and sparring mitts. Having received tens of thousands of sparring punches (often not aimed accurately) in his mitts, his right shoulder finally gave way, and needed surgery. His ingenuity and knowledge of the sport led to his invention of the BOXMASTER and FIGHTMASTER training machines. Both comprise twelve padded punching targets about twice the size of an average hand, mounted on a sturdy frame and weighted down. The targets are arranged for the standard boxing punches: straights, hooks, upper cuts and body rips. The machines are strong enough to withstand a professional boxer in full flight; the BOXMASTER is the heavy-duty version for serious boxing gyms, and the FIGHTMASTER is a lighter-weight version for studios and home use. After ten years of design and development, Rai had the patented machines working like he wanted, and was successfully manufacturing them in China and selling them around the world.

In about 2015, Rai was attending a trade show in Europe, and he came across an academic physiotherapist from Portugal, Josefa Domingos, who was using a FIGHTMASTER machine to train PD patients in boxing. Rai was delighted to see his invention being put to such worthy use, but noted that Josefa hadn't quite set up the machine correctly. He was worried that incorrect use of the device could lead to injury, and was concerned that it would be very difficult for physiotherapists to provide expert tuition in boxing techniques. He also knew that BOXMASTER machines had been purchased by gyms in the USA where the Rock Steady Boxing program was used for large numbers of patients with PD. It planted a seed in his mind, that started to grow when he saw a poster at an airport in the US. It was a picture of Michael J Fox, advertising his foundation with a slogan, 'Out Fox PD.' Rai immediately thought of 'Out Box PD,' and how this might be done with his knowledge of movement and the training machines.

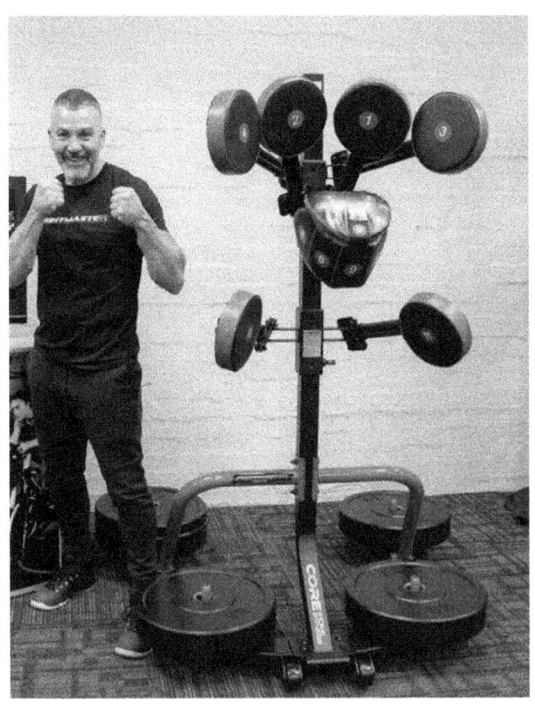

*Rai Fazio and his FIGHTMASTER boxing training device*

## Meeting Rai

I met Rai for the first time towards the end of 2019 at the Perron Institute. Rai's long-time friend Denis McInerney was an acquaintance of Steve Arnott, the Perron Institute CEO. Denis helped to arrange the meeting. Living in Perth, it was difficult not to have heard of Denis. At one time in the 1990s, his radio advertisements for his Ford car dealership seemed to be playing continuously. The catchy jingle joked that 'Denis', 'Mac' and 'Ernie' were giving you three for the price of one. Denis is definitely a larger-than-life character, kind, jovial and extremely generous, and he helped to finance Rai's movie. I admit I had some reservations before the meeting, not about Rai, but about the concept of boxing. As a neurologist it felt a little uncomfortable being associated with a sport that was linked to head trauma. The Perron

Institute has an entire scientific team devoted to head injury research, so from an institute perspective this could be a bad look.

Any concerns I had about this issue were completely erased at the first meeting with Rai and Denis. Rai described his story, and evolving interest in using boxing training to help train PwP; there were tears in his eyes – and mine! He immediately offered to train me and see if we could come up with some sort of program to help patients.

## Preparing FIGHT-PD

The main goal Rai had was to help people with PD. I naturally shared that, along with my vested interest to help myself. As a clinician though, I knew that despite the best of intentions, interventions for medical illnesses are complicated. Over many years I have seen vulnerable patients desperately grasp at therapies offered unscrupulously by people focused only on financial gain. Even well-meaning individuals who support unproven therapies can do PwP a disservice by wasting their time and money.

All these reasons were behind our desire to run a clinical study, and to create an exercise program. A fundamental issue was to ensure safety. A big part of that was around correct training technique. How much training and how intense the training could be, in conjunction with medication also seemed like an unanswered question. Finally, how to create an optimal program that people with PD could complete, needed to be addressed and of course, what everyone wants to know, does it help? Doing all these things with scientific rigor would bring validity and integrity to the program. The best-case scenario would be to have a validated program that health insurers could fund as a therapy for PD.

Before we could address any of these questions, I needed to learn a lot more about boxing training, and also to do it myself. Rai and I started in early 2020 with a few simple sessions covering boxing basics. I quickly came to realise that boxing is an enormously technical and skilled sport, with huge demands on strength, aerobic fitness and concentration. What immediately made sense to me was that the posture and movements necessary for boxing were in almost every way the counter of the abnormal postures and impaired movements in PD. In PD, there is a tendency to stoop forward with flexion of the spine and arms. In boxing, one needs to stand up straight, and when making a punch (particularly jabs and straights), extend the arm fully beyond the target. The PD movements are small, weak, slow and imbalanced; boxing's must be large, strong, fast and with excellent balance. An education in neuroscience is not required to suspect that boxing training sounds like a perfect exercise for PD. Thankfully, I didn't have to build my fitness from scratch, because even Rai's basic warm up (well before putting on the gloves), is quite an athletic challenge. When I was doing a lot of running, it was usually large volume and low intensity. Sometimes, when I was getting serious for a race, I'd include some interval training of 200 metre sprints up a slight incline as part of my program. Rai had me doing star jumps, twists and lunges, so I got the feel for high-intensity exercise again – and enjoyed it.

It took time to develop strength in the hands and wrists, and they ached for a while, but it was fun to learn something I had never done before. During this period, I spent a lot of time reading about exercise in PD, and was particularly interested in a review article[7] about boxing for PD. It was by an academic physiotherapist in Melbourne, and leader in exercise for PD, Megan Morris. It was an excellent article but left me dismayed to see how sparse the available evidence for the effect of boxing was; just thirty-seven patients studied in two quite old papers[8,9]. It then struck me; here was an opportunity for this deficiency to be corrected. Reading this paper, and realising this gap in knowledge, was highly motivating for me. With Rai's knowledge, the assistance of the Perron Institute and my own personal insights, it seemed this was a clear pathway of research opening up for us. I could barely contain my excitement, and was soon making notes, as plans and thoughts swirled in my head.

Around this time another distraction was looming. The disturbing reports about COVID-19 were becoming publicised. The horrendous scenes from Italy of body bags remain blazed in my memory.

During these early stressful days of the pandemic, Rai and I pushed on with training. We were able to continue sessions using Zoom. In fact, the first time either of us used Zoom was to train during COVID lockdowns. Rai had kept just ahead of the COVID-19 wave, having been in both China and the US a few months before the outbreaks in each area occurred. Now, his usual busy travel schedule was suddenly becalmed. After an initially frantic organisational time, I also found myself with more time than usual. Patient numbers were initially down in the hospital; people were staying away from public hospitals. Perth and Western Australia was to become one of the world's regions least affected by COVID-19 in the first year. It's geographic isolation, with oceans to the west, south and north, a huge desert to the east, and a limited number of borders and entry points, was key to keeping COVID out. The state government pursued a strong policy of border restrictions which further cemented this advantage. There were cases of people returning from elsewhere, but very limited community transmission. Like Rai, I usually travel a reasonable amount; typically, one overseas trip per year, usually for medical conferences, and two or three interstate trips for meetings and conferences. All this travel came to a halt, and after the initial flurry of work related to preparations, and reorganisation within the hospital, I found myself with some extra time. I used this to work with Rai, to train myself and to develop plans on how to apply what I was learning to others with PD.

Rai has dozens of different workouts, and many years of experience teaching people of widely different abilities how to box. It soon became apparent to me that punching was only a small part of the sport, with the ability to move and maintain balance and posture being critical to get into a position to make a punch, and avoid being hit. I had already started to feel the balance problems that come with PD, so it was exciting to specifically train to develop skills for improving balance. We built up the training steadily, in much the same way Rai would train someone to build up for a competitive fight, usually over about twelve weeks. I would eagerly take notes during and after each session, dripping sweat onto the pages of a note book that I had been cramming with thoughts and ideas. It seemed to me that there really weren't many exercises that I, or other patients with PD, couldn't attempt. The only exercises that really troubled me, involved moving the head from a low position to a high position; this created transient light headedness. We decided to avoid this, since orthostatic hypotension is a feature of PD, and complication of some medications. This refers to a fall in blood pressure when standing. Usually it is defined by a fall in systolic blood pressure (the top number) by more than 20 points. This results in reduced blood flow to the brain, creating the feeling of faintness. We certainly wanted to avoid that, and the risk it brings of passing out and injury. As I progressed through the training, I concentrated on undergoing everything we would put patients through in a trial setting. I learned to warm up, cool down and manage the aches and pains of training, and how that interacted with the aches and pains of PD rigidity. I also learned to time my PD medications to optimise my mobility for training sessions. I made sure I did a lot of stretching, and extra yoga. The goal for my training was not only to get myself in shape, but also to learn as much as I could to help design a clinical trial for PD patients. As my training progressed, I could feel the benefits coming on. Even though I had muscle soreness for a few hours after each session, I felt I could walk more easily. My arms steadily gained strength, and I could actually see my right wrist and forearm muscles building up, whereas before they were withering. At some point in the training, Rai added in what he calls 'flurries'; a 10–15 second burst of punches (usually uppercuts), as fast and as hard as you can go. He counts them down so that if you are flagging, you can push on to the end; like a swimmer pushing hard to get to the wall, or a runner to the line. These bursts were challenging, but seemed to coincide with further improvement. In effect, this was high-intensity interval training, or HIIT. This comprises a burst of near maximal effort for a short period of time (10–60 seconds), followed by a brief period of rest, before repeating[10].

Crucial to the trial design process, was the knowledge and expertise of Dr Travis Cruickshank and his PhD student, Mitchell Turner. Travis is an academic exercise physiologist based at Edith Cowan University in Perth, with specific expertise in using exercise as a treatment in medical conditions. I had known Travis for several years, and we had always been looking for research collaborations between his team and the Perron Institute. His work on exercise in patients with Huntington's disease was impressive, and his knowledge of exercise as a therapeutic intervention and how to study this was exactly what Rai and I needed to develop our plans. Travis already knew of Rai and his FIGHTMASTER machines; he was also familiar with Josefa Domingo's work[11]. Travis knew very well how to prescribe and measure exercise. This did not appear to have been done, or at least described well, in any of the previously published papers on boxing training for PD.

One of the key things we aimed to achieve with FIGHT-PD was to quantify the amount of exercise being done. This is a key component of any study where exercise is used, and the best studies of exercise for PD using treadmill walking[12], stationary cycling[13], and brisk outdoor walking[14], all measured heart rate (HR). If boxing training was to be compared with these, we felt it was important to measure HR, and we wanted to see if this seemingly simple thing could be done. I'm not sure why this hadn't been done in the other small studies of PD. Perhaps there were concerns that the vigorous body movements performed during boxing training would make monitoring difficult. I tried a popular brand monitor with a chest strap that recorded HR and sent results immediately to my phone. To my delight it was easy to use and didn't impair movement at all.

The other way to measure exertion is to use a Rating of Perceived Exertion (RPE) scale. One of the most commonly used scales was developed by a Swedish researcher named Borg[15]. The most frequently used version of this scale ranges from 6–20, with 6 being sitting, resting quietly, and 20 being maximal effort. High intensity, or the 'red zone' is 17–20. Training above 17 will have you gasping for breath and struggling to talk. Travis and Mitchel instructed me in the use of this scale while I was training with Rai, in preparation for its use in the study. The RPE scale can also be used to try and quantify the cognitive difficulty of a task, and is denoted RPME, with M standing for mental.

A vital part of a clinical study is to clearly define the questions you are asking. Our basic question was simple: was it feasible for people with early PD to do the FIGHT-PD training program? In the simplest terms, it was about ensuring their bodies would hold up without injury. I was keen to push them hard, perhaps as hard as they could go, under close supervision. I had experienced first-hand how good I felt after Rai had pushed me, and wanted to know if other PwP could feel the same. Additionally, I was impressed by the experimental animal data and Jay Alberts'[5] work with cycling regarding the benefits of 'forced exercise,' where pushing exercise above the comfort zone was the real key to improvement. Any experienced sports coach knows this, but applying it to people with PD, even at an early stage, could be opening new ground. I was certain our participants could achieve high-intensity training, which is usually defined as exercising at a heart rate of more than 80% predicted maximum for age[10]. My interest was to see if we could get participants to do high-intensity interval training (HIIT). I hadn't always been a proponent of HIIT, especially because of my work in stroke, as I knew that large variations in blood pressure can trigger stroke or heart attacks in predisposed individuals. In order to minimise these risks, we screened participants very carefully, which included proper cardiac stress testing, undertaken by a well-regarded cardiology laboratory.

HIIT was exciting to me, but for Travis and the exercise physiology team, it was a bit old hat, with the sports literature already well acquainted with the topic. They were keen for the study to integrate some ideas they had about designing exercise therapy into blocks, where the focus could be shifted from demanding physical tasks to more challenging mental tasks. There is strong neuroscience theory behind the neurorehabilitation strategy of dual tasking[20], where participants are required to learn and perform tasks while exercising; an ideal way to stimulate the brain.

By the end of 2020, the protocol for our first study had come together; we actually made twenty-eight different versions, with frequent changes, as our plans evolved, before we submitted it to the University of Western Australia's Human Ethics Committee. I love acronyms for studies and in less than a minute, **F**easibility of **I**nstituting **G**raduated **H**igh intensity **T**raining; FIGHT-PD came to mind. It also tied in with Rai's FIGHTMASTER machine. In November, Rai, Travis,

Mitch and I presented our plans for FIGHT-PD to a group of about sixty PwP and their relatives. I have given hundreds of lectures, conference presentations and public speeches, but rarely have I been more excited and engaged with an audience. Without rehearsal, our talks all blended together, and it struck me that Rai, Travis and I all had links that made it seem like fate had joined us together to do this.

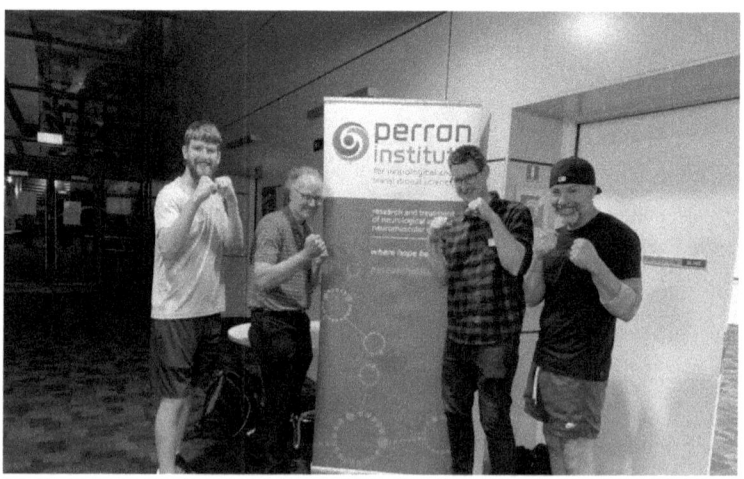

*Left to right: Mitchell Turner, me, Travis Cruickshank and Rai Fazio after our public presentation of the plans for the FIGHT-PD study. Hosted by Parkinson's WA November 2020.*

The response to our plans for FIGHT-PD was enthusiastic, with many more people volunteering than we could include. This created the difficult situation of having to tell people that we didn't have a place for them. I am much more accustomed to clinical trials being undersubscribed, so I hadn't expected to be having these awkward conversations. We kept a master list of everyone who had indicated interest in being involved, and in the interests of fairness I methodically worked down the list in chronological order, screening people for involvement in the study. We wanted to be sure everyone was suitably fit to handle high-intensity exercise, so one of the key things was for all potential participants to undergo a cardiac stress test. One man, who mentioned he'd had some vague chest heaviness when hiking a small mountain, had some serious ECG changes on the test and was found to have a worrisome coronary arterial narrowing that was promptly treated with stents. He was very disappointed to miss out on FIGHT-PD.

It took less than a month to have the ten participants for FIGHT-PD selected and prepared to start. There were six men and four women, which is about the gender balance typical for PD. The average age was sixty; about half were still working, the others were retired or semi-retired. Most were already quite fit and active, and three were fairly regular golfers.

## FIGHT-PD works for me

As we developed the FIGHT-PD study further, my own fitness and strength began to noticeably improve. This gave me great encouragement to push on and do the study. By early 2021, I was probably not quite as fit as when running marathons, but I had a more varied fitness regimen which included two boxing sessions per week, two or three sessions of yoga per week, two rounds of golf per week, and a baseline minimum of 15 kilometres of brisk walking per week. My 2021 New Year's resolution was to do 100 push-ups per day; I was fanatical about that, and after a few weeks I could really feel the difference. The arm strength from boxing and push-ups also helped my golf game, adding extra distance to my driving. Matthew, our younger son, was home for a couple of months from December 2020. He's a vegetarian, so we ate a mainly vegetarian diet for this time and I lost some weight. Additionally, I gave up alcohol completely. Like many university students of the 1980s, I could party hard. I recall drinking more than a dozen beers on a weekend night and still being able to get up early the next morning and play competitive golf. During my working life I had never been much of a drinker; the constant demands of call and need to be available always tempered the amount I consumed. I always had a worry about alcohol triggering migraines as well; on occasions, just a small amount of red wine would do this. As my PD developed, my lack of sense of smell had removed the pleasure of wine anyway. At some stage towards the end of 2020, I had maybe two or three beers one night, and next day felt absolutely dreadful. I had a mild hangover, combined with the start of a migraine, and then a PD 'off' period. I had been starting to get some 'end of dose' symptoms and on this day I had them badly; my walking felt like wading through mud. It really scared me because it made me worry that in the future I might be like that all the time. Following this episode, I concluded that it didn't make sense to drink alcohol when I had a neurodegenerative condition. A while later, I developed some difficulty with swallowing as part of PD, and needed to pay attention to posture when drinking fluids, otherwise I'd trigger a bout of coughing. The last thing I needed was to be intoxicated and breathe wine into my lungs! This further encouraged me to avoid alcohol. Several months alcohol free, further contributed to some weight loss, so I was fitter and leaner by the middle of 2021 than I had been for many years.

## PD you can't see

COVID brought long overdue medical hygiene practices into sharp focus. The hospital policy quickly changed to 'bare below the elbows' for all clinical staff. After years of wearing a suit and tie, I was pleased to make the change to short sleeves. Besides, buttons and ties were becoming problematic as my dexterity diminished. Because of this change in wardrobe, there were staff at work who had rarely seen me in anything other than a suit and tie but who could now see my arms. My forearm muscles had become well defined, and I was happy to have regained the strength I had previously been losing. As a result of my reduced stress and enthusiasm for the FIGHT-PD study, I appeared better than I had for some years; even my neurologist said, 'You don't look like someone who has PD.' When he said that, I suddenly appreciated what I had long been aware of in some of my own patients; looking well externally is of no solace if you are struggling on the inside. Some of my most upset and depressed stroke patients were those who had no visible external signs of neurological deficit. Well-meaning family and acquaintances often comment on appearance, and almost always, patients will say they are fine, allowing internal frustration to build. Some PwP (including myself at times) find this difficult to deal with. The emotional reaction can be complex. If you are feeling vulnerable and a little paranoid, the thought bubble can easily be 'don't you believe that I have PD?'. There can be a sense that observers can't know how much effort is going on inside you to maintain what appears to be normal function. Neither can they see the fatigue, interrupted sleep, lack of sense of smell, muddled thinking, difficulty concentrating, anxiety, apathy, tendency to feel extremes of cold and heat, dizziness, sudden urges to use the toilet, constipation and many other non-motor symptoms that plague us with PD. I'll digress with a metaphorical situation that might illustrate for those without PD why it may appear that sometimes PwP appear completely normal.

I want you to imagine a scenario. A pair of identical twins, neither of whom has PD, are at an airport. They are the same weight, have the same fitness level, and have both had the same amount of sleep and breakfast. They have a very long walk to the gate and they come across a travelator, or 'moving sidewalk' as they are called in North America. Let's call 'twin A' the twin who continues to walk on the normal surface, and the other, 'twin B,' the twin who steps onto the travelator. Unfortunately, twin B' has accidently stepped on the wrong lane, which is moving in the direction opposite to where they are walking. Twin B takes up the challenge of keeping up, despite the need to walk against the movement.

Initially, twin B can keep up, but because of walking against the movement, needs to move faster and use more energy than twin A. If twin B is very fit, this might be maintained for a while. Aside from twin B's arms and legs moving quickly, the two twins still appear much the same. As they continue for longer, twin B starts to fatigue and falls behind. Twin B stops for a brief moment and falls way behind. Their names are called over the public address system because the flight is leaving now. Twin B puts in a concerted effort, catches up the ground and arrives at the same time as twin A. Now twin B does look a bit different; breathing heavily, sweating and flushed, and with hands shaking when holding the boarding pass. Twin B collapses into their seat feeling fatigued after the extra effort, and shortly after take-off falls asleep, exhausted.

This is what it looks and feels like for many people with PD. In summary:

- We can keep up, but it takes more effort.
- It can be difficult to see the effort, especially if the face is expressionless.
- If we stop moving, we go backwards (that is, the progression continues).
- With great mental effort we can catch up (and maybe get ahead).
- After covering the same amount of distance as others, we can begin to look tired.
- We are prone to fatigue and need to rest.

Although I was looking well, I was acutely aware of how much effort I was putting into staying that way. I was keeping up my now quite complex exercise regimen, and having to be quite vigilant about taking the L-dopa, which was typically giving me about two and a half good hours before things started to deteriorate. Night times were becoming especially challenging. For years I've had to get up once or twice a night to urinate, and now, in the early hours, doing that in the off state was starting to become tough. The combination of postural light headedness, bradykinesia and painful rigidity, were all nightly reminders that the PD was still there and very real. (I sometimes imagine this is a preview of what it might feel like to have a ninety year-old body.) I often awoke with vivid nightmares that made it very difficult to get back to sleep. On the days when I played golf, I sometimes marvelled at the transformation I would undergo. Waking two hours before tee time, barely able to move, I'd take a Madopar immediately, followed by caffeine, a hot shower, and stretching. I tried to delay eating food as long as possible to optimise absorption of the Madopar. I'd arrive at the course (a five-minute drive) one hour before tee time, and then run through a modified version of my boxing warm up, doing the rotational exercises focusing on shoulder and trunk movements. Another coffee while hitting forty warm up balls and I'd be ready to go, with nothing to suggest that two hours before I was a decrepit, creaking mess, barely able to get up.

So, when everything was going well, my PD was quite invisible to others. Apart from Kirsten, no-one ever sees me when I'm 'off.' It would only be apparent if I was really tired, unwell with a migraine or had missed a dose. I was taking five or six Madopar per day, and some long acting Madopar HBS at bedtime, but I needed better symptom control overnight. In early 2021 I added in Safinamide (Xadago). This reduces the breakdown of dopamine, effectively prolonging the effect of the Madopar. My neurologist, who was not a movement disorders subspecialist, hadn't prescribed this before (and neither had I), and it wasn't being used much in Perth. I read as much as I could find about it, and listened to an extremely informative webinar hosted by one of my colleagues from Adelaide who had done some training with me in Perth. It seemed the Spanish had a lot of experience with this as an add-on agent to L-dopa, reducing 'off time.' There was also a suggestion it might reduce dystonia related pain, which I was especially interested in to help with my troublesome right foot.

My right foot continued to worsen through early 2021, but it became apparent it was not just the PD; there was a mechanical component to the pain, and after a while it became clear to me that I had plantar fasciitis. To some degree I'd made the mistake that PD patients and their doctors can make of blaming a new symptom on PD, when in fact something else is going on. A few months before, I'd missed the bottom step of a set of stairs in our house while barefoot, landing heavily on my heel. It wasn't particularly painful at the time, but gradually I noticed an aching throb, which seemed to peak after exercise, and was prominent at night. It started to become a real problem after golf. I'd shower, have lunch and then, when getting up to move again, find that I could barely walk because of the pain. For the rest of the day, I'd struggle to get around, and if my PD meds were a little late, the whole thing would compound. New shoes, pain killers and stretching didn't seem to help. In March 2021, my annual golf trip was to south west Western Australia, rather than interstate, because of COVID. I managed to get through the five rounds in five days, and played reasonably well, but I took a lot of pain killers and did plenty of yoga and stretching. After this burst of golf, the symptoms were getting out of hand; I needed some help. I obtained an x-ray of my foot, just to make sure there was no obvious bony pathology, then saw a podiatrist. She was fantastic. I saw a little smile coming across her face as I described my symptoms; the smile I also get when you hear a patient history and you know what is going on and realise that you can help. She had plenty of knowledge and numerous practical tips to help treat plantar fasciitis. After a couple of weeks it started to become manageable. I began to use a motorised cart to get around the golf course, and was delighted to be able to complete a round with a manageable level of pain. There was a COVID-19 lockdown in Perth in April 2021, so instead of playing more golf, I did a lot a writing, yoga and binged the specific foot exercises. That was a turning point to getting it under control. It remains in the background, but I now know how to manage it. The experience further enhanced my respect for my allied health colleagues.

# FIGHT PD begins – the early rounds

Meanwhile we were getting closer and closer to starting FIGHT-PD. Another short COVID lockdown reduced access to the Edith Cowan University campus with a subsequent two week delay. In mid-May 2021 we were finally ready. One Saturday, Rai, Travis, Mitchell and I spent the whole day setting up the gym with FIGHTMASTER machines. I calculated that between three of us, we moved 1,800 kilograms of equipment that day. Despite taking care of posture and position, I wound up with a sore back but the pain was surpassed by the excitement of being on the cusp of the project we'd been planning for more than a year. The following Wednesday evening, we held a two-hour introductory session for our first cohort of ten PD participants. I couldn't help but be excited and a little manic, having been awake since 3.30 am, my head full of thoughts. There was much to do. Rai personally adjusted each machine to match each person's height and we marked correct foot positioning on the floor. Mitchell expertly sorted out the IT issues, linking everyone's phone to the heart rate monitors, and sorting out access to the surveys and scores to be at each workout session. I called the PwP participants 'PD-FIGHTERS.' They seemed excited like me, but I was concerned we would be overwhelming them. Any fear of this was dispelled when we started our first proper workout session on Monday 24 May.

There was a lot for us all to take in and pay attention to on the first night. Rai was eager to ensure that everyone got attention and good instruction. I was terrified that someone would hurt themselves, and was particularly worried about a couple of the older participants. I've been the principal investigator on many clinical studies before, shouldering the weight of responsibility for adverse events and pretty much anything that could go wrong. That was usually in the setting of studies of medication, where a side effect would typically occur slowly and I might learn about it after a few days. FIGHT-PD was different, something could happen at any second. Right before my eyes were ten participants, potentially one fall away from a broken hip. However, I could see the impact of Rai's instructions on balance technique having an impact in real time. By half way through the third workout, I could already see improvements in the participants I was worried about, and I could start to relax a little. After the first week, they were glowing; sleeping well after the exercise and with no reports of injuries. Almost all of them seemed invigorated. The buzz in the group was palpable. The research team was working very hard to manage the many details of the study, but we could all see this was a great project with potential to help all the participants and create new knowledge. Rai very wisely had arranged for a friend of his, Raz, to make video recordings of all the FIGHTERS at several time points through the study; this included a short interview and action footage.

## FIGHT-PD– the middle rounds

FIGHT-PD continued through the winter of 2021. The study was organised into three training blocks, each lasting five weeks, with the fifth week being a rest week. Each week consisted of three one-hour workouts: Monday and Wednesdays at 6 pm and Friday mornings at 7 am.

The first block was designed to be an introduction to boxing techniques, development of fitness and strength, and familiarisation with the assessments. I was thrilled to see the drills that Rai and I had developed, put into action. Travis, Mitchell and their students utilised their expertise from previous exercise studies by comprehensively measuring the efforts of the subjects using numerous scales and scores and continually monitoring heart rates.

Each workout was a big commitment for participants. While some lived close to the university campus, several had to commute for more than an hour, often during peak-hour traffic. Before each session there was a sign in, and completion of online surveys to measure pain, fatigue and sleep. Any niggles or health issues were reported, and Rai and I made sure to accommodate for these during the session. Sometimes this meant adjusting technique, sometimes an exercise was modified or skipped. The heart rate monitors were fitted and linked to phones, wrists strapped and final adjustments to the FIGHTMASTER machines made. Every participant had a specific machine allocated to them, with the height carefully adjusted and markings made on the floor and the punch pads.

The workouts all started with a systematic loosening of the body from top to toe, starting with arms being held 90 degrees to the sides of the body, then elbows flexed and extended with increasing vigour for about a minute, with this being done in both a side-to-side and an in-front position. This very simple exercise, which Rai's father used to start loosening up for boxing training, encourages arm straightening, which counters the tendency PD has to flex the arm. Further exercises concentrate on 'waking up' the shoulders, and then gradually working down the body, including some shadow punching to get ready. It was nice to fall into a routine with these movements, and within just a few workouts, there was a definite sense of the whole group falling in sync within a few minutes of the start of the warm up. After this, Rai guided the group through a series of boxer's movements, which aim to keep the boxer light on their feet and avoid getting struck. These movements are excellent for balance and strengthening core and leg muscles, and also seem ideal for helping people avoid falls. I am sure these skills have helped me adjust rapidly when I have tripped, averting several accidents.

After about ten to fifteen minutes of this, the group was usually looking warmed up and ready to go. Sometimes we included a short jog when we had enough space, before adding in a few exercises designed to crank up the cardiovascular workload, including twist jumps, lunges, and my favourite, star jumps. I'd never done star jumps before meeting Rai, and when he and I were training together I think Rai was surprised at how many I could do. (In fact, I surprised myself at the start of our training in 2020 by completing two minutes of this very demanding exercise.) I was pleased that I still had a good standard of cardiovascular fitness, despite the fact that I couldn't effectively run anymore. On one occasion I was really flying with the star jumps, and was very disappointed to twinge a calf muscle – a reminder to take care, and a warning that it doesn't take much to injure an ageing body.

The FIGHT-PD warm up is as much exercise as a full workout in other PD programs such as PD Warrior – and that is before throwing a single punch. There is no doubt these rounds of punching on the FIGHTMASTER machine are the highlight, and the most fun, but the warm up is important to prepare for this. Even though the warm up and boxer's movements components of the workout provide an excellent cardiovascular challenge, it's amazing how much additional conditioning benefit is derived from the boxing section of the workout. (During a three-week break around Christmas 2020, I kept up my cardiovascular fitness, especially the high intensity elements and yet, upon return to the boxing, I struggled after just two or three rounds, whereas before I was getting through six.) Rai points out that each punch is like lifting small weights, and each workout has hundreds of punches. I recall the feeling of my wrists and arm becoming stronger, and the Fighters could feel it too. We could see them getting stronger and moving more freely. A couple of them initially had the classic, short shuffling PD gait and slow movements, and it was a thrill to see this improving before our eyes. Even though the study was structured and designed to measure feasibility and safety, rather than a before-and-after comparison, we did endeavour to measure this with a standard scale used in PD studies, and with videos performed at the start and then at various points through the course of the study.

After the first one-month block of FIGHT-PD we had planned a one-week break in order to give the participants a rest, enable recovery from any developing niggles and to catch up on any missed workouts. A COVID-19 lockdown extended this break to almost two and a half weeks. Thankfully, we were able to conduct several Zoom-based workouts to help keep up the participants' form and fitness. Our initial experience in doing Zoom sessions proved very valuable.

It was great for the group to reconvene for the second block. Now the Fighters were confident with the techniques, it was time to push them. They all knew when we consented them that this section of the study was going to be tough, with the intent being to escalate the dose of exercise. The study team remained vigilant, looking for the emergence of pain, injuries or fatigue. The group surpassed expectations; only four workouts (in the entire study) out of the 360 possible, were missed due to minor injuries in two participants. I accompanied the Fighters, doing most of the workouts as well as overseeing the group and watching out for injuries. I liked to do the workouts as often as possible; it meant I had good idea of what they were feeling, so I could be vigilant if it was going to be too much.

During this middle block, we were able to crank up the music accompanying the workouts. In the first block, we had to keep quiet for many of the workouts because student exams were underway in a nearby part of the gymnasium complex. With this restriction gone, Mitchell supplied a 'boombox' and Rai the soundtrack, which was heavy on classic 1980s hard rock, especially ACDC. This was the music of Rai's and my teenage years, and most of the Fighters loved it too. One of the highlights towards the end of the program came from one of our Fighters, a retiree who had previously worked in radio, and had been a DJ. He is a Scotsman, so one day he wore a kilt for the workout. The ACDC classic, *'It's a long way to the top,'* contains a bagpipe section, during which time he really rocked the kilt. The addition of music to the middle block really seemed to make the exertion easier. I vividly recall one Friday morning when the group was just buzzing along at a very high rate of exercise in time with the music. I was also training with them, with dopamine, caffeine and exercise levels all optimised; it was the best I had felt in years; almost elated. Most participants reported similar windows of exercise-induced wellbeing, even euphoria. This is likely due to the effect of various metabolic changes triggered by high-intensity exercise, which might favourably impact on PD.

We minimised the planned rest week between the second and third blocks because the threat of further COVID related lockdowns worried the team that there would be an interruption to the study, which would be difficult to make up. In the final block, we eased back on the cardiovascular intensity and introduced some mental challenges to the workout. It seems that the combination of cardiovascular load with cognitive challenge is likely to be the best way to stimulate the brain in both healthy and diseased brains[16]. Again, the Fighters handled the workouts well, although it seemed they actually preferred the higher-intensity workouts. Our initial plan was to study twenty participants, but with all the COVID related delays and alterations, along with the intensity of the study, we all decided to leave it at ten. It was always going to be a small study, but what it lacked in numbers was made up for by the amount of detailed data and experience we obtained.

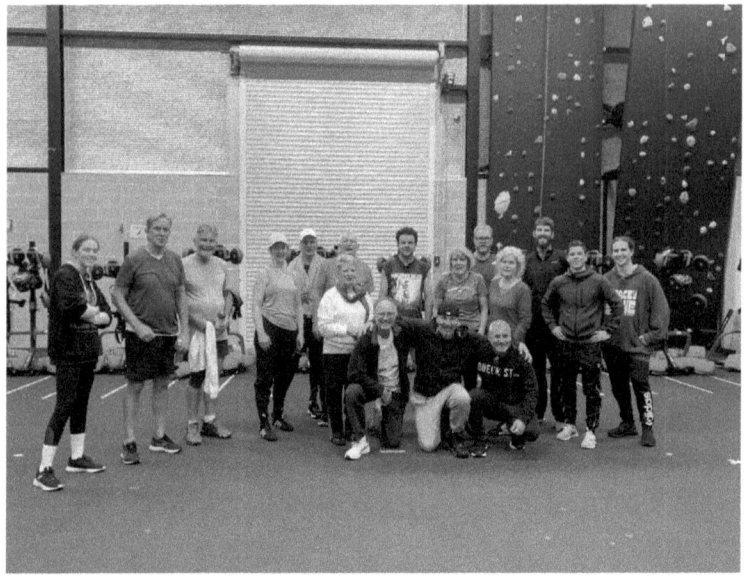

*The FIGHT-PD study team and participants in the gymnasium at Edith Cowan University.*

## The final bell and beyond

In early September we finished FIGHT-PD. The final workout was quite emotional. There were speeches and thanks. There were some tears, but overall, there was a great sense of accomplishment and a definite sense that this was not the end. I told the Fighters that I very much hoped that the fitness, strength and confidence they had developed would continue for the remainder of their lives. The whole study was exhilarating, and Rai, I and the other team members were proud of what we had achieved. We only had to look at how well the Fighters were moving, and how trim they looked, to see how far they had come. There were a few final study details to finish, including a formal exit interview with me at the Perron Institute, and a repeat of the Unified Parkinson Disease rating scale (UPDRS), to be compared with one performed at baseline.

Shortly after the final session we had a get together at a bar, with almost everyone involved, including all the Fighters and their partners. It was a surprise to see everyone smartly dressed, rather than in training gear. To anyone watching us, it would have appeared to be just a group of friends or colleagues out enjoying a drink and a get together, not a group of people with PD. During this event, Raz took each Fighter aside, and made a final video recording.

Rai and I were very mindful there could be a let-down if the Fighters just stopped training. Rai and his wife Bella were extremely generous in giving the Fighters some time at a small gymnasium Bella was renting, to continue training on Tuesdays and Saturdays. Between six and eight of the Fighters attended these sessions, and I attended most of the Tuesday evenings which became not only training, but also catch up sessions. For me, it was like going to a patient support group. This was no longer the FIGHT-PD trial, with the formality and stress placed on both Rai and me, it was a group of friends (who happened to have PD) getting together to work out and feel better. I think we all understood how Rai's workouts could make us feel better, even if we were having a bad day. My role as researcher and doctor was no longer so important; I was just working out, and I enjoyed seeing the group.

During that time, we had a lot of work to do: collating the data, starting the write-up and considering how we could apply what we had learned to more people with PD, and perhaps undertake more research.

## FIGHT-PD results

The main objective was to determine if the vigorous non-contact boxing exercise program could be done by a group of people with early-stage PD and completed safely, and if measures of exercise could be recorded. We achieved all those objectives. All participants completed the fifteen-week program and 348 of 360 (97.7%) possible workouts were completed. Only four of those 348 were missed due to minor injury related to the intervention.

We recorded and reported the logistical details describing the time for ethics approval, the screening and recruitment process, resource utilisation and costs. All this is extremely valuable for the planning and design of future studies.

We recorded heart rate data from 302 out of 348 (86.8%) sessions. Most of the data missing was because of failure of the phones to synchronise with the HR monitors, or participants simply forgetting to turn their program on. We had a huge amount of HR data which we may be able to analyse in even more detail, but the main conclusion was that all subjects were able to train at a high intensity (>80% of predicted HR maximum) for at least thirty minutes, three times per week.

Questionnaires tracked measure of fatigue, sleep and pain over the course of the study. We were surprised to find that fatigue and sleep both improved, and there was no change in self-reported levels of pain.

The other question that participants and the public want answered, is whether or not it makes a difference. I went to great lengths to always emphasise that FIGHT-PD was never designed to scientifically demonstrate a statistically significant difference caused by the intervention. Firstly, there was no comparison group (also called controls) – a group of individuals with PD, matched by similar baseline characteristics (age, gender, stage of PD) who underwent standard care involving their usual program, or perhaps another form of exercise program. (Another valid way to make an analysis of a treatment benefit would be for participants to be their own controls. This would involve a staggered program where assessments are done at set time periods across a set interval while doing their usual exercise program; this would then be repeated while undertaking the FIGHT-PD program across the same amount of time.) Next, the assessment tool we used, the Unified Parkinson's disease rating scale was administered before and after the program by a neurophysiotherapist trained in the administration of the scale, but not blinded. (In order to avoid bias, the optimal arrangement is for the UPDRS to be administered by staff who are independent of the study, and don't know if the participants have had the intervention or not.) Finally, our small number of study participants meant that we would never have the statistical power to make an analysis of any therapeutic effect. It is common in early phase and feasibility studies to measure a treatment effect anyway, with a view to using this information to form the basis for calculating what the size of future studies would need to be in order to show statistical significance. Nine out of ten participants showed an improvement in their before and after UPDRS scores.

A free copy of the FIGHT-PD paper[17] can be downloaded from the *PM&R (Physical Medicine and Rehabilitation) journal* at https://doi.org/10.1002/pmrj.12986

The **FIGHT** is not over

# FIGHT-PD – the documentary

Rai and I had both wanted to give all the participants in the FIGHT-PD study, video documentation of their remarkable progress. All the Fighters were filmed at various points along the way. Rai's experience with movies and television, and connections in the film world, ultimately produced a 45-minute documentary covering the FIGHT-PD study. It included some background on how we met, how it all came together and highlighted the amazing way it evolved. We hired a medium sized theatre for a private screening of 'FIGHT-PD: The Story. A documentary showing how 10 people with Parkinson disease are fighting their way to better health using exercise.' The participants, their partners and a select number of invited guests brought the crowd number to about eighty. It was at a tricky time during the COVID pandemic, because government-mandated protocols had to be strictly followed. There was a possibility that the city could go into another lockdown period, so we rushed to present this during a stable gap. It was a memorable evening.

## UK Trip – COVID knocks me down

We'd planned a trip to the United Kingdom as soon as our son Matthew moved there to study in mid-2021. At that stage, travel in and out of Western Australia was tightly controlled by COVID restrictions. When Matthew left, Perth International Airport was like a ghost town, and the customs officials had to call Canberra directly to ensure all his paperwork was correct. He'd been studying in Canberra for the past four years, so Kirsten and I were familiar with him leaving, but this was different; it was to the other side of the world, with uncertainty about how long he would be away, and when we could visit.

By late 2021, there were glimmers of hope that travel was opening up, so when tickets became available for the resumption of the direct Perth to London flight, we were quickly onto them. We made plans for a long stay, from the end of May to the end of July 2022. I stopped taking on new patients at the start of April, in order to avoid having unfinished issues while we were away. By this time, I finally started to believe we were going to be able to travel; the UK COVID restrictions were loosening, and a version of the pre-COVID world was returning. Kirsten and I had both had three COVID vaccinations, but before our departure in May, we were not eligible for a fourth; we were not old enough or sick enough to qualify.

The last month before leaving was hectic. I was keen to write up the results of the FIGHT-PD study and have this submitted to a journal before we left. It was helpful to have a deadline because I may otherwise have kept revising and re-writing it indefinitely. Finally, on 24 May 2022, we were in the air, on the seventeen- hour flight to London. As I dozed fitfully, I could hear someone nearby with a persistent dry cough, but there was nothing to be done. We arrived at Heathrow feeling reasonably well. We kept masks on in the terminal, but were in the minority and on the Underground, very few people wore masks. We made our way to Kings Cross, where we rented a tiny two-bedroom apartment; a central location where we could recover for four days, and do some tourist things before embarking to Dublin for a tour of Ireland. At least that was the plan.

For the first two days we were fine, and we did a surprising amount of tourism with zest and enthusiasm, including the London Eye, Westminster Abbey, the National Gallery, the British Library, and a classic double-decker central London bus tour. On the third day, Kirsten decided to stay in the apartment and rest. I was still keen to go out, and even started the day doing a high-intensity workout in a small nearby park – including star jumps and shadow boxing.

The National Hospital of Neurology and Neurosurgery was nearby; a highly respected institute where many Australian neurologists had done the additional training, like I had done at the Mayo Clinic. It was interesting to ponder if two years in London as opposed to Rochester would have shaped my career differently. While contemplating this, I wandered a little further to the British Museum. Kirsten was not a great fan of natural history museums (she much prefers art galleries), so this was a good chance to explore this solo; I was particularly keen to see the ancient Egyptian collection. While there, I had an abrupt onset of fatigue and lethargy. I recall coming out of the bathrooms on the lower level and looking upwards at the long curving stair case, thinking it looked like a mountain. It was a distinct wall, more abrupt, and quite different to what I'd felt in any of the six marathon races I'd run. I knew it signified something bad, but at that point wasn't quite sure what. Slowly, I trudged back to the apartment. Kirsten had been having a restful day, but was quite fatigued; she assumed that the effects of jet-lag were catching up with her.

That night I woke with a fever, chills and sore throat. This was not a challenging diagnosis; the rapid antigen (RAT) COVID test I took just before midnight lit up positive. I e-mailed Kirsten a picture of the test to greet her when she woke. She took her RAT test the next morning with a matching positive. Despite both of us feeling dreadful, we realised there was a need for a confirmatory PCR test, to permit ongoing travel and insurance. Conveniently, there was a COVID testing facility within 300 metres.

The next few days were an exhausting blur. I felt like I had every symptom of all the colds or flus I ever had, all bundled into one. I never felt in danger, but I had a strong understanding of how a frail, unvaccinated person could have died of this. Despite being prepared, having brought supplies of analgesics, anti-inflammatories and decongestants with us, I was shocked to experience waves of fatigue early on. Within the first day, we both realised that we'd not be fit to travel to Dublin as planned. We managed to extend our stay in Kings Cross for a single day, but needed to find another place. The Queens Platinum Jubilee celebrations were to begin within a week, and accommodation in London was tight. Eventually, we located an apartment in Maida Vale, West London. The next challenge was to move across London on day four of COVID infection, while still feeling dreadful. This proved to be the epic low point of the trip. We assumed we were still infective, so we took great care to avoid possible contact with others. We arranged for a black London Cab for the transfer across town, and were pleased to learn that apparently the NHS had used them for patient transportation because of the separated compartments between driver and passengers. This was not the major issue during the hour-long trip we took later than day.

One of my COVID symptoms was mild diarrhea. In the apartment this was not much of a problem, although I already had a little pre-existing 'faecal urge' likely related to the PD, which meant I often had to go quickly to the toilet. When we boarded the taxi, I had thought my bowels were all under control, but within a few minutes I suspected I was terribly wrong. There was no doubt I could not hold on for the rest of the journey, and we were going to have to stop. I don't think the taxi driver understood what was happening when we pleaded for him to stop and let me out. Difficult seconds passed while Kirsten tried to explain the urgency of the problem. Things were desperate, as I eventually I burst out of the door, onto a busy Euston Road. We were near the British National Library, which we had visited two days ago and I knew there were public toilets in the lobby. Thankfully, I knew in which direction I needed to dash. I managed to adopt a gait and facial expression that apparently clearly conveyed to motorists and pedestrians an unspoken message that at any second my bowels were going to explode. I must have been quite a sight; dishevelled and with an ungainly 'anal squeezing/ PD gait' and a look of desperation. It felt like the longest two minutes of my life as I finally made it into the lobby. I hurried by a room containing rare documents such as sketches by DaVinci and an envelope with original lyrics written by the Beatles. I made it just in time. I'd thought that an episode of embarrassing faecal incontinence was almost inevitable, so there was a huge sense of relief. After cleaning up with what seemed like wafer-thin scratchy one-ply, the next task was to find Kirsten and the taxi. Thankfully phone tracking and Google Maps came to the rescue. The remainder of the transfer was less eventful, although a slight rumbling recurred with about five minutes to go.

The next task was unanticipated; an apartment on the fourth floor and no elevator; sixty-four stairs! About a decade earlier I'd run up more than fifty flights of stairs to the top of one of Perth's tallest skyscrapers in a fundraising event for Multiple Sclerosis. That now seemed simple compared to the task of dragging our suitcases up all these stairs with our bodies drained of energy by COVID. After the ascent we were sore and tired, but not short of breath – Kirsten rightly noted that COVID had not got into our lungs. We collapsed onto a sofa, utterly exhausted.

The apartment was fabulous, with two bedrooms, two bathrooms, a large living area and a generous balcony overlooking a busy intersection in the middle of Maida Vale. From the balcony, to the left I could see Wembley Stadium, and to the right I could almost make out Lord's cricket ground. It proved to be an ideal place to recover – in fact Kirsten remained in the apartment for a full seven days before venturing down the stairs, mainly to avoid having to climb back up again. The large sofa was a fantastic place to rest and watch endless BBC repeats of classic 1980s rock hits and then the Queen's Jubilee celebrations. We could hear the crowds amassing for this, and we got a great view of the aircraft flyover with their coloured exhaust trails. We didn't have the energy to join in the celebrations and were not keen to spread COVID to thousands of people. Even though the COVID isolation laws had ceased in the UK some months before (February 2022), the public health advice still recommended isolating for seven days, as did our own conscience. I was feeling a little better by then and had begun short exploratory walks in the mornings. I started to resume exercise gently. My bowels were a slight problem, and I wondered if it was a lingering effect of COVID, another infective process, or possibly the entity of post-COVID immune colitis. The other concern was about absorption of my medications. Apart from trying to maintain hydration and avoid spicy foods, I didn't think there was much more that I could do, and hoped it would settle down soon.

There was still 'holiday work' to attend to, most notably rebooking our planned tour of Ireland. There were a few days where we both felt well enough to do some tourism before a new wave of COVID fatigue crushed us both. It was like nothing I'd ever experienced before. With

PD, I'd experienced end of dose 'wearing off,' which felt like wading through mud in an emotionally fragile state until the next dose kicked in. The COVID fatigue was much deeper, more overwhelming and more persistent, and I became worried that my many years of work on fitness and strength would evaporate. I began to use hand grip springs to keep my wrists strong; squeezing out sets of 100 several times per day. Any time I sat on the sofa I did a set. I also re-started my regular push-ups, which pre-COVID had included at least 100 per day. I was cautious, only doing about 20% of the volume of my usual exercise at less than half intensity. Kirsten suffered similarly, and for the remainder of the trip there were times when it would hit one or both of us in a bout of global lethargy, superimposed on a baseline of tiredness.

We eventually made the trip to Ireland after sorting out the necessary clearances and insurance issues. The post-COVID fatigue was still there, and we had to ration our energy carefully. Thankfully, we were able to catch up with Matthew in Cambridge and then travel north to Edinburgh. I was able to attend the final round of the Scottish Open golf and then the Monday practice round of the British Open at St Andrews, both unseasonably hot days for Scotland. We made our way back to London by train, and were there for the hottest day on record, 21 July. On that day, we met up with some friends from Brighton, who very generously took us to lunch in a fabulous Chinese restaurant on the thirty-third floor of the tallest building in London, The Shard. We'd first met them on a tour of China in 2018, so a Chinese banquet in commemoration of that seemed fitting. We had remained in touch intermittently ever since, but the subject of PD had never really come up. Kirsten had mentioned it in correspondence in the weeks previously, in order to avert the chance of any undue over-sympathetic reaction that would detract from the fun. As it turned out, our friends were to see first-hand what PD could do to remind me it was still there.

Usually, when we venture out somewhere Kirsten will have a couple of spare Madopar tablets with her. This time she didn't have any, possibly because our routine was a bit different to usual – we actually dressed up a bit, knowing this was a fancy restaurant. It was also historically hot for London, to the point where the train system was failing and we were a bit pressed to get to our planned meeting point at the bottom of the Shard building on time. We were feeling a bit frazzled by the time we made it there and somewhere in the excitement of our greetings and getting through the airport-like security required for entry, I managed to lose my supply of Madopar. I wasn't too worried at first, but then realised that with less than an hour till my next dose and with a long lunch and journey home ahead of us, things could become challenging. Our hosts were charming, and after some great food, spectacular views and what was apparently good wine, we said our farewells and headed back on the Underground to our apartment in Hackney. I'd gone more than six hours without a dose of Madopar and the results of this inadvertent experiment were worrying. My right leg was dragging and my right hand cumbersomely slow and tight. I was grateful to get back to the apartment for a dose of Madopar, but it didn't help much. My discomfort was compounded by the heat in the flat so we left the apartment a night earlier than we'd paid up for and caught a cab to Heathrow and an air-conditioned hotel. We checked in and were relieved to find ourselves in the last hotel room of the trip. After a long day in the heat and getting behind on my L-dopa dosing, I was getting one of those emotional downers that can come when in a PD 'off state.' As I dragged myself into the bathroom, the churning intestinal strife I had experienced before the Ireland trip welled up again and this time I didn't make it, soiling myself less than a metre from the toilet. I slumped down on the floor, sobbing and exhausted, comforted by Kirsten and the thought we'd be home soon.

## Back to Perth

It was a relief to be back home towards the end of July 2022. There was no pressure to return to work, although I went in and collected the usual large pile of papers that accumulates when one is away for a while. When we organised the trip I had factored in a possible fourteen-day period of COVID related quarantine for overseas travellers returning to Western Australia. This was no longer required, so it left a convenient passage of time to get my cataract surgery done. With this completed, the whole world seemed so much brighter and my decades of wearing glasses was over. Something still wasn't quite right with my vision, with the balance of the new lenses not quite aligning. This made catching up with my backload of correspondence quite difficult.

## Fatigue and depression

The fatigue that I had felt since COVID was still there, and several times per week there would be an overwhelming wave, when I just had to rest. I could only manage a full day's work if I had a short nap at lunch time. Even on those days, I was only seeing a small number of private patients and going to the Perron Institute. Somewhere among all of this, the fatigue became combined with intense periods of emotionality and distress. I suddenly felt frail, and old, and had lost enthusiasm for the future. I'd even lost energy for golf. There were occasions where I found myself lying down, drained of energy, and crying. It was time for more help. Again, the diagnosis was pretty straightforward. I'd become depressed, as do at least 50% of PwP.[18]

After a visit to my neurologist, we decided to start Lorazepam (a short acting Valium-like drug) at bedtime to help me get off to sleep, and hopefully reduce the intrusion of prominent dreams. I also raised the questions of starting an anti-depressant and of seeing a psychiatrist or psychologist. My neurologist supported the idea of an anti-depressant, but was lukewarm on the value of psychiatry in my situation. The Lorazepam did seem to help, reducing the dreams and dream enactment, although after about a month they returned, but with less intensity. It also helped me to get back to sleep more quickly when I awoke (as I usually do) about two hours after going to bed.

The anti-depressant we chose was an older drug, Sertraline, which I had prescribed for my own patients many times. I didn't start it immediately, because I wanted to double - check a potential interaction with the Safinamide, which was also an anti-depressant, from a class of drugs called MAO-B inhibitors. Older forms of this class of drug, when combined with other drugs or certain foods could potentially cause serious side effects such as the serotonin syndrome and dangerous elevations of blood pressure. I had already done a lot of reading about Safinamide when I started it, and the local pharmaceutical representative for the company marketing it had helpfully provided me with detailed information. I'd also watched two webinars hosted by some leading Australian movement disorders specialists, and featuring some colleagues from Spain, where it has been a popular drug to add in to L-dopa when motor fluctuations appear. A moderate sized case series [19] (collection of patients with thorough description of their characteristics documented and evaluated to expand the knowledge of a condition) showed no major side effects when Safinamide was added to Sertraline, but there seemed to be nothing about adding Sertraline to Safinamide. I even checked this with a direct enquiry to the pharmaceutical company scientific team, who gave a cautious, conservative response. I thought it would be a good idea to monitor my blood pressure closely, so I purchased an automated blood pressure machine. I also started using this in my private practice, instead of the manual sphygmomanometer which I was finding a little difficult to use because of diminished dexterity in my right hand. Many years ago, before my exercise revolution, I'd had slightly elevated BP in the order of 130/90, so the concern was that this new combination could raise that to problematic levels. I need not have been worried. Ever since my PD diagnosis, all of my BP recordings had been 120/80 or lower, and as previously explained, at times I had symptoms of low BP, especially when playing golf in hot weather. After making some baseline recordings of BP, I started the Sertraline without any problems.

Unlike my own neurologist, I was more enthusiastic about psychological help, and Kirsten was also keen for me to get some extra assistance. I contacted a colleague who is both a clinical psychologist and neuroscientist, and with whom I had previously done several research projects. We agreed that we knew each other too well for me to become a patient, but they were able to provide the name of another psychologist who turned out to be an excellent choice. I was relieved to set up an appointment, even if it was to be in a couple of months.

The other aspect I started to attend to was the future structure of my work. To some degree I felt daunted about continuing clinical work.

The stress of acute stroke consultations was particularly challenging. For decades, acute stroke had been 'my thing'; in fact, I was one of the first neurologists to push the 'time is brain' treatment attitude in Perth. Despite having seen thousands of patients, many of them initially in the emergency department or CT scanner and very early in the course of their stroke, this remains a tough and stressful form of medicine. I considered that I was now too physically slow and not mentally sharp enough to do this. As I noted before, I didn't want to put patients at risk, and I was also increasingly mindful of how stress would worsen my own symptoms. The fatigue and vision issues were also affecting my ability to read and keep up with the latest in the literature. I felt I was no longer as up to date as I should be and was starting to lose some confidence in my clinical skills.

## Changing gears and direction

Around this time, I happened to assist a number of my patients with insurance and income protection claims due to their PD. This typically required detailed reports including dates of consultations, test results, letters and answering many questions about how PD was impacting their work performance and other aspects of their lives. Their situations were quite similar to my own, and the subsequent payouts provided some financial security. This encouraged me to look closely at my policies and begin an application. I had looked at this before, just after the diagnosis, but because I was still working at full steam it appeared I was not eligible. In fact, in 2019, bolstered by the early improvement following the commencement of Madopar, and the extra work of being head of department, I had one of my busiest and highest earning years. It had been steadily downhill since then. I now felt morally justified in making an insurance claim, especially when I read that specialist physicians' peak earning years were in their mid-fifties; I had also paid many thousands of dollars into these insurances. Despite this sense of justification, it was still a confronting task to see on paper the end point of the main part of my career.

I also spent some time reviewing articles about the effect of PD on working and early retirement. One study[20] noted that at five years after diagnosis, only 50% of people with PD were still working; 2023 was going to be my fifth year. I gradually became accustomed to the idea that it was time to phase out the clinical work and begin to let people know I was retiring and not accepting new patients.

I began organising referrals for my private patients to other colleagues and seeing some patients for the last time. This was emotionally draining for me, as some patients were quite upset. Many could not understand why I was retiring. I needed to allocate double the usual time for a patient appointment in order to explain things and say goodbye. I found it useful to use an analogy with Ash Barty, the top Australian tennis player who in 2022 shocked the sporting world by retiring at the peak of her game and as the reigning Australian Open champion. Like her, I wanted to get out while still at the top of my 'game,' particularly before I started making mistakes. One unexpected joy, was a sense of fulfillment referring some patients on to neurologists in private practice who had been my trainees. It gave me a sense of satisfaction that my mentoring and teaching efforts were having tangible benefit.

A key reason for ceasing clinical practice was the stress of the responsibility and decision-making. I always had the feeling that the buck stopped with me, even though in most cases I would be sharing the care of an individual patient with other doctors, and always their GP. As I began to feel more tired and frail, this became too great a burden. The fear of making a mistake started to worry me and added to my insomnia.

In contrast, the research work that I was doing always involved a team, so I could be replaced if I became unwell. This gave me confidence to focus on my roles at the Perron Institute for Neurological and Translational Science and at Argenica Therapeutics. I feel very fortunate to have been able to shift my career in a different direction. If I hadn't developed PD, I may not have had the chance to participate in some very exciting research.

By the time I got to see the psychologist, I was feeling a good deal better. In retrospect, I suspect I was more depressed than I realised. It is likely that a combination of factors contributed to the improvement, including the medication and work decisions to cut back and reduce the stress. I felt relief knowing that I had an extra support for the future, with further psychology appointments now booked for regular reviews. That was a good thing, because the next few months were to involve some extraordinary challenges.

## 2023 – a rollercoaster of events

The next short-term goal was to prepare for a golf trip to Melbourne beginning the first weekend in March. Each year, since 2016, I've travelled east with a group of long-term golfing friends to play five consecutive days at some of the top courses in Australia. I consider this week away a highlight of the year. Most of us are serious, single-figure handicap golfers who gear up our games for the tour. I've found it very useful to have regular goals like this to focus my exercise regimen. To play my best golf I need to maximise my aerobic fitness, strength, flexibility and balance. All these are important to counter PD. A quiet, positive mindset is also very helpful. I almost enjoy the preparation as much as the event, a bit like in my days of running marathons, when the training made me feel great. During my time working in neurorehabilitation, the allied health staff taught me a lot about goal setting and how important it is for neurological illness. Fighting PD is a bit like being an athlete training for the Olympic Games. It's a long-term business, and you can't possibly keep training hard all the time. To make it manageable, it needs to be broken down into smaller chunks, with motivational events along the way. The training needs to incorporate lighter days and weeks to allow for rest and recovery. It also needs to be flexible, in order to manage injuries or illness.

I played reasonably well on the 2023 tour and had a great time with my friends; the inevitable late nights and altered diet tested my stamina, and by the end of it I was quite wiped out.

It was always a little tough to get back to work the week after a golf tour, but 2023 was a bit easier because of my substantially reduced schedule. Just prior to the tour, I had seemed to be getting more 'wearing off' of my L-dopa, typically at about 2.5 hours. Earlier in the year, I'd started taking some extra-long acting Madopar in the mornings, and when I was playing golf. I was finding that my right foot was again dragging, and my right hand was up to its old trick of sticking during certain movements, such as getting a golf tee out of my pocket, and when trying to place a ball on the tee. I would take the regular Madopar a little earlier than usual in order to keep my movement enough to get through a round of golf. I even started taking an occasional rapid acting L-dopa preparation for times when I felt I was getting really stuck. After the golf trip, I continued on this slightly higher dose, which I felt I needed to get through a day of work, and also in order to feel I had sufficient leg movement to be able to drive home in the evening. During the golf tour, I'd noted the emergence of what was likely 'peak dose dyskinesia': Quite reliably, forty-five minutes after a dose of regular Madopar, my right shoulder would begin to shrug and twist involuntarily; it was only subtle, and lasted just a few minutes. I'd also noted a tendency for my right foot to twist and turn in when I spent more than about 30 seconds standing still over a putt. I could diminish this by either taking the shot more quickly, or adjusting the position of my right foot.

A brief, post golf tour 'funk' didn't last long; within two weeks I was back in Melbourne, attending a medical education event hosted by some of Australia's leading experts on PD. This was the first time since the COVID pandemic that I'd left Western Australia to attend an in person medical meeting. I had forgotten how nice it is to see old friends and colleagues at such meetings, and how the whole educational experience is richer than anything that can be presented on-line. These meetings covered a variety of topics, including how best to manage the more advanced stages of PD. What I took away from the sessions was a better appreciation of the role of deep brain stimulation (DBS), notably its beneficial impact on quality-of-life measures, and the fact it has fewer side effects than the other advanced therapies, such as gastro-intestinal

L-dopa gel and subcutaneous L-dopa or apomorphine. It affirmed my impression that there are not many people with PD who undergo successful DBS and come out saying, 'I wish I hadn't had that done,' or 'I wish I'd waited longer'; almost universally the feeling was the opposite. This was perhaps akin to not deferring the commencement of L-dopa, in order to not miss out on its benefits. There appeared to be a 'window' which could pass, after which time DBS was less favourable; for example, if cognitive decline from other medical issues developed.

I returned to Perth with a lot to think about, and a feeling that my PD journey was about to enter a new phase. My decisions over the last few months to slow down my clinical work, seemed to be vindicated and I was now thinking it was almost time to have a consultation about DBS. I wasn't to know that the remainder of 2023 would be so eventful that any thoughts of DBS would need to be deferred. It was a good thing I wasn't overloaded with work, because this time (from May to October) would comprise a rollercoaster of highs and lows.

First, some of the highs. Shortly before my trip to the PD meeting in Melbourne, in early March I received a very official looking e-mail from the office of the Governor General of Australia. The subject was regarding acceptance of a proposed award: a Membership of the Order of Australia (AM) in the King's Birthday Honour's list in June. The implication was that this was virtually a forgone conclusion. However, there was a process to go through, including answering some questions – and keeping quiet about it for the next three months! To be awarded an AM in recognition of my achievements in medicine and neurological research was an amazing honour. I'd always viewed these awards as going to celebrities, prominent sportspeople, or professionals coming to the end of long careers. The latter certainly seemed to be my category.

In mid-April I received an e-mail from the editors of the *PM&R Journal*, notifying me that the FIGHT-D paper had been accepted for publication. Not only was this a joy, it was a great relief. While I knew that it would eventually get published, to prepare a fourth submission would have been very tough. This also gave the FIGHT-PD exercise program some extra credibility, as Rai and I slowly worked to start making FIGHT-PD a program that could be accessed by many more PwP, and marketed.

Shortly following this, I was notified that I was a finalist in the Western Australian of the Year (WAOTY) awards. Several months previously, the Perron Institute had put me forward as a candidate. I didn't give much thought to it at the time. The annual event was in its fiftieth year, with numerous categories, including the professions (the one I was in), community, arts, indigenous, sports and young Western Australian of the Year. Just over 150 nominations had been received and about fifty were shortlisted. This was narrowed down to three finalists for each of seven categories, with a winner in each — and also the overall winner, The Western Australian of the Year. This was to be announced at a gala event on the first weekend in June. It was another great honour to be in the running for an award that had been won by some very prominent people. Regardless of whether I won or not, it was also a great opportunity to publicise the work I had been doing in stroke, and then more recently in PD. One morning I arrived at the Perron Institute to learn that one of the young scientists, Adam Edwards was also named as a finalist, in the Young Western Australian of the Year category. It was then that I fully embraced the excitement of all this. Adam was part of the scientific team I had been collaborating with on neuroprotection. His expertise was in a condition named hypoxic ischaemic encephalopathy (HIE) in newborns. This occurs when the infant brain does not receive enough blood or oxygen. There are numerous scenarios when this may occur, notably in premature infants with lung problems. Amazingly, Adam himself was born at twenty-five weeks and was at great risk of HIE. His work was now focused on experimental models of HIE, with a plan to use the same peptide that I was involved with for adult stroke. For about the last six months I had been meeting with Adam to help create a strategy for progressing his work in the laboratory into clinical trials. Our work with the same medication for adults was several years ahead of Adam's, but it was exciting that everything we were learning in applying this treatment to adults, would assist with the work in infants. I don't think two Western Australian of the Year finalists had ever come from the same institution in one year, so everyone was proud and enthusiastic.

There was a very busy three-week build-up to the WAOTY awards. One of the first things was a detailed interview and filming session, over about three hours. This was to produce videos for publicity and for the gala event. My interview covered a lot of ground including the clinical and research work I'd done with stroke, and more recently the PD work, especially FIGHT-PD. Peter Coghlan* (see special note), my famous patient who had a 'locked in syndrome' stroke kindly came in to participate in the interviews and filming. Rai also came in for the exercise work, and this included me gloving up and doing some boxing for the cameras. Over the next two to three weeks, there was extensive publicity, including television, newspaper, radio and on-line exposure. Independent of this publicity (and a few days before the announcement of the WAOTY finalists), Rai and I appeared on local television news with the results of the FIGHT-PD study. The following day I caught the train down to Bunbury to stay with my Dad and visit Mum on Mother's Day. I knew the WAOTY publicity would commence with a big article on the finalists in the Saturday newspaper and I wanted to be there when Dad opened the paper and saw it. It was a great thrill for us both. The television news covered it that night (making it my second appearance on the news in three nights), and then the Sunday newspapers ran it again. Over the following two weeks, there was further coverage in various media. When the WhatsApp group for my medical school group exploded with comments, it was all getting a bit much. Over the years I'd had more than my share of media exposure, but this blitz was starting to be embarrassing. There would be more publicity closer to the event, but first my roller coaster of 2023 was about to plunge downwards again.

# PD when you can't see

On 1 May 2023, I met with my neurologist for a general check-up, and to discuss a plan to approach the emerging issue of motor fluctuations. We also chatted about considering a visit to one of the movement disorder specialists to discuss DBS. The plan was to add in an old drug, Amantadine, which has been around for decades. Its initial use was as an anti-viral drug to treat influenza A infections. It also may have a mild alerting effect through amphetamine-like chemical pathways. In PD, it has a role when motor fluctuations appear, especially dyskinesia. I had not prescribed it very much myself, but my neurologist was very experienced in its use, and at the recent meeting I attended in Melbourne, it had been given quite a positive critique. It certainly sounded like a good plan, but I did want to thoroughly check the possibility of interaction with my other medications, particularly the Safinamide. All appeared fine and safe, so I started it a couple of days later, eager to see if it would make a difference; an alerting effect would be a great bonus to quelling the dyskinesia. Additionally, there was an outbreak of Influenza A in Perth at the time, so possible protection from that would be a most welcome advantage.

On the second day, I noticed a strange feeling in my left eye. There was some slight shimmering in the vision, and a weird sense of fullness in the eye, almost like there was some water on the surface. The next day this continued, and there were some 'flashers and floaters,' briefly obscuring my vision. I then very nearly fell into the 'Dr Google self-diagnosis trap.' I had been aware that Amantadine could possibly exacerbate glaucoma and was a bit concerned about that possibility. I also found reports of a rare complication of Amantadine; corneal oedema. What I was feeling in my left eye certainly felt like fluid, so I was hopeful that simply stopping the Amantadine would be the solution. The problem was, the reported cases of this had all involved chronic usage of Amantadine over many months or years; not just three days. Momentarily, I thought I could write myself up as a case report of 'very early onset corneal oedema associated with Amantadine.' I was soon to learn I was very wrong.

On Sunday afternoon we went to the movies, and I realised my vision was obscured. To make matters worse, I then developed a migraine, including the visual aura that often accompanies migraine. The brightness of the screen and the loudness of the movie left my head throbbing and gave me a sense of nausea. I staggered out of the cinema leaving Kirsten and James to watch the end. There was no quiet in the foyer so I went outside and sat by the car. Having emerged from the darkness of cinema into the natural light of the outdoors, I was shocked to note there were gaps in the vision of my left eye. This was not like any migraine I'd ever had, and I knew I needed to have this evaluated. My main worry was glaucoma, and I could get that looked at by going to an emergency department. My heart sank at the prospect of going to any emergency medical facility late on a Sunday afternoon, when typically the backlog of medical emergencies is at a peak. I started making some phone calls from the car park while I waited for Kirsten and James to see the end of the film. I spoke to an ED colleague working at one of the private hospital emergency departments, who suggested they weren't well equipped to deal with such ophthalmic issues, and it would be tough to get access to an ophthalmologist. He advised going to the nearby public hospital (SCGH). It never occurred to me I could have called my friendly ophthalmologist who I had been seeing for my glaucoma for many years. The migraine pain was settling, but I was a little nauseated, and I don't believe I was thinking terribly clearly, my post migraine brain being somewhat stunned. The SCGH Emergency Department was surprisingly quiet and I was taken quickly to the eye room. One of the senior emergency nursing staff who had expertise in eye reviews assessed me. I recounted the history of glaucoma, the new PD medications, and my concern that my intra-ocular pressures could be raised. The nurse quickly and efficiently measured the pressures (which were normal), and did a 'slit lamp' examination (to look at the surface of my eye); no corneal oedema. I had wrongly assumed I was going to be seen by one of the doctors to finish the assessment, but that was not on their agenda. I was reassured that it wasn't glaucoma, and I knew it wasn't a stroke, but there wasn't a clear diagnosis. I could feel the migraine coming back, and suddenly just wanted to go home, with a new plan to call my ophthalmologist first thing in the morning. I was exhausted by the time we got home, and for once slept quite well. Kirsten was working early on Monday, and I reassured her I had a plan and would sort it out. I actually had two ophthalmologists I could call; the cataract specialist who had operated on me the previous year, and my long standing glaucoma specialist, a colleague from my year of medical school. He listened to my history and within seconds recognised it could be a retinal detachment; he suggested I get to his office quickly.

When I put the phone down I felt like an idiot. Through a combination of having a little bit of incomplete knowledge, use of Dr Google, fixation on a limited differential diagnosis and addled thinking due to migraine, I had missed a potentially sight-threatening diagnosis. I hurriedly packed a bag including an ample supply of PD medications, and began to fast, knowing that I'd likely be heading for an operation at some stage. To complicate matters, my ophthalmologist was at his 'south of the river' office that morning, so I had to catch a taxi across the city through peak-hour traffic. It was a long journey, during which I kept testing the vision in my left eye which was now highly obscured. And all the while feeling like I had made a blunder that might delay sight saving surgery. I was to learn later that while this is an ophthalmological emergency, it's not in the same realm as the emergency of stroke where it has been estimated that every minute of delay can see two million brain cells die[21]; I'd spent most of my career working with that mindset. Nonetheless, it was a further dent in my increasingly wavering confidence in my medical skills. If I couldn't make a diagnosis in myself, how could I confidently do so in other people?

My ophthalmology colleague's examination confirmed his suspicion of a spontaneous retinal detachment involving the macula (area for central vision). Myopia (short sightedness), prior cataract surgery and age, were the three identifiable predisposing factors. A bit depressing to have 'age' on the list for this condition, which is actually an example of your body falling apart – even more depressing!

So the diagnosis was made, but an epic day was far from over. I was referred to a retinal specialist who was to become my third ophthalmologist – I have more eye specialists than I have eyes! This office was back on the other side of town, so another taxi ride was required. Kirsten met me for the second appointment, which included making arrangements for admission to the eye hospital for surgery that evening.

The surgery to repair a detached retina is remarkable. One of the components involves the injection of a sulphur containing gas bubble, which makes up the volume of the ocular fluids that are lost with the surgery, gradually dissolving over two to three weeks as the fluids re-accumulate. My understanding is that it also has a role in the acute post-operative phase to keep pressure on the freshly lasered retinal surface, keeping that in place. Depending on the location of the detachment, you need to lie in a specific posture to ensure correct positioning of the gas bubble. In my case, this was face down, in the prone position.

The awkwardness of this position, combined with a slightly 'off' PD-state due to a long gap in Madopar doses, a hospital gown that kept trying to strangle me, a tangled non-functioning intravenous line and the stress of the whole day all made for an absolutely wretched night. I was still wearing my work pants when I got back to the ward face down, and with all the issues described above I was pretty much stuck. Kirsten has not lost her general nursing skills, and somehow managed to replace my work pants with more comfortable pyjamas when I elevated myself on my toes for a few seconds. The PD 'off' was thankfully averted by Kirsten facilitating my overdue Madopar dose, and some of the rapid acting formulation. Kirsten later told me the nurses seemed horrified at how slow and frail I was at that time, and wondered how much help I was getting at home– the assumption being that I always needed help getting dressed. They were probably incredulous that I could still be working as a specialist. This was a rare occasion when I really did look like I have PD, and it is not pretty. In fact, most nights when I shuffle to the toilet at about 2 am and then struggle with insomnia, I feel what I assume it's like to be over eighty years of age; at least based on descriptions my dad gives. That night after the eye operation was a much more profound version, and a horrifying glimpse of a possible future time.

There was a suggestion at some stage that I could go home at 11 pm, and then attend the surgeon's office at 8 am next day. On this occasion, my addled, post-anaesthetic brain made a good decision; 'No way!' Even when the Madopar kicked in, the thought of staggering down to the car, then getting up a few hours later to come back across the city for the third time in twenty-four hours almost had me in tears. I finally got some sleeping tablets, discarded the strangulating hospital gown and had the IV line taken down. I then did some yoga breathing techniques to eventually settle. I vividly recall trying to calculate how many breaths I needed to take before the morning came. The combination of yoga breathing, an overdue sleeping tablet and finally getting the bed organised, resulted in some sleep at last; at about 5 am. I then had less than ninety minutes of surprisingly deep sleep before I had to be up in time for the discharge procedures and for Kirsten to pick me up and take me to the eye clinic where the surgeon was to check on me.

The post operative check showed that everything was as expected. The surgeon double-checked I wasn't due to fly anywhere in the near future; the gas bubble can be disrupted by depressurised conditions. He assured me there would be steady improvement. I'd already been looking at articles which noted that involvement of the macular region (as in my case) predicted incomplete recovery. I thus entered a limbo where it was uncertain what would ultimately happen to my vision. With the bubble still present, it was quite a strange sensation. It's like having a spirit level in your eye, with a fluid level that jiggles around as you alter position. The other analogy is that of wearing swimming goggles and positioning yourself so that part of your vision is below the surface of the water and part above. Reassuringly, as the 'meniscus' began to sink, the emerging vision appeared to be quite clear.

This period of rapidly changing vision was quite disconcerting, and made me a little nauseated. I found that by wearing a patch to block the distorted vision from the recovering eye seemed to help a bit; although the pirate jokes quickly became old! While legally I could have driven using the vision of the good eye, I actually didn't feel confident to drive. It would have been nice to rest a bit and give myself a chance to recover, but the opposite occurred. The surgery was done on the Monday night of a crazy week of activity. The publicity related to the Western Australian of the Year Awards was in full swing, following on from the publicity regarding FIGHT-PD. I ended up doing a television interview from our front room that Thursday because I didn't feel like moving from the house.

## Too much of me on TV

On Friday 2 June, I attended the Western Australian of the Year Awards ceremony at the Crown Hotel and Casino, as a finalist. Kirsten, my elder son James and my father Kevin attended as my guests, along with several of my closest colleagues from the hospital and the Perron Institute. I was thrilled also to have Rai Fazio and his wife Bella at the table; their first big night out since becoming parents. This was a glitzy, black-tie event with over 600 attendees – all manner of dignitaries, including the governor and numerous high-level politicians and former premiers. For Mark McGowan, who had announced his shock retirement as the premier of WA a week before, this was his last public event. It was an Oscars-like award presentation with seven categories, each with three finalists, as well as the overall winner; the Western Australian of the Year. Each category had several minutes of video footage of the finalists, made from the filming sessions we all did a few weeks before.

This year's winner was Gina Rhinehart, billionaire mining heiress, philanthropist and the richest woman in Australia. It was an honour to be among all these famous people, but it was certainly not my comfort zone. The best part was being able to share it with my family, friends and colleagues, and in particular to give Dad some joy, in what had been a tough few years with mum's dementia and his own health issues. Kirsten and I stayed in the hotel that night, and then escaped to the tranquillity of a yoga retreat for the weekend, where thankfully no-one recognised me. The awards were a thrill, but emotionally exhausting. The yoga retreat was a great way to calm down and refocus. I found the two solid days of yoga made a meaningful improvement in the flexibility of my legs, particularly the right leg which had become increasingly tight. This yoga-induced serenity didn't last very long. During the following week, the King's Birthday Honours Order of Australia list was publicised. After keeping it quiet for three months, the recipients were announced. This resulted in a further appearance on TV news as well as newspaper coverage. Over the next week there were many texts, calls and e-mails from friends and colleagues from all around the world offering best wishes and congratulations. This had a far wider reach than the WAOTY, and was probably a more satisfying type of recognition, although, once again, I felt I was getting too much attention. When I participated in the TV advertisement for the Perron Institute a couple of years before, strangers sometimes approached me at the local supermarket asking, 'Where do I know you from?' This was starting to happen again, with my face recognisable, but not famous enough for people to know who I was. I was grateful for an opportunity to escape from this for a short time.

## A brief escape

My next adventure, at the end of June, was a trip to Barcelona to attend the Sixth World Parkinson's Congress (WPC). The WPC is a unique event with about 4,000 attendees all involved with PD, patients themselves (or their relatives), and researchers and clinicians. Unlike other conferences I have attended where just a few patients were present, there were probably as many people with PD as any other group, at this meeting. I met three other doctors with PD, and I'm sure there were many more. I also attended a number of presentations on exercise. It was great to finally meet Josefa Domingos, the physiotherapist whom Rai had met all those years ago, and to give her a copy of the FIGHT-PD paper. I also met Dr Cormac Mehigan. He is a consultant emergency physician working in Limerick, Ireland, a PwP and keen golfer. We'd previously exchanged e-mails when he very kindly made contact with me after reading my article[4] in *Practical neurology* in 2020. He and Kevin Fitzpatrick were key people in the establishment of the Irish Parkinson's Golf Network, formed several years ago. They have about fifty members now, and they meet up for a game together every few months at various courses around Ireland. Cormac outlined his plans for a bigger event to be held in Ireland specifically for PwP and asked if I'd like to participate; 'Absolutely, yes,' was my immediate response. I was also interested to learn about other sports recently embraced by PwP, including pickle ball and table tennis.

One of the sessions was a round table discussion about exercise. The important take-away message was that most people with PD want some guidance on establishing an exercise routine, rather than being left to their own devices.

I presented a poster[22]; *A neurologist with PD: what I've learnt about being a patient, and a person with PD. Can communication with doctors be improved?*

It focused on my experience with the early stage of PD just after the diagnosis, and presented perspectives from both angles. I made suggestions on how communication might be improved. A European survey[23] revealed that only 49% were satisfied with the initial diagnostic consultation, so there is a lot of room to do better. The poster could have been perceived as being somewhat critical of my neurological colleagues; it also made suggestions on how PwP could do some simple things to improve the interactions. Although a reasonable amount of people seemed to be viewing it, there was not as much reaction or interaction as I had hope for. It struck me then that my situation placed me in a curious limbo. I was neither fully a person with PD, nor fully a health specialist because I had biases and ideas from both sides. Strangely, I felt a bit lonely despite being in a huge crowd and I was glad to be going home soon.

## A new opponent

I recovered reasonably well from the travel, and had given myself plenty of time before restarting my now reduced work commitments. Having this extra time may have saved my life because it meant that I promptly attended to some routine health checks which, in previous years, I had tended to drag my feet on. The first was the bowel cancer screening test (that starts at age fifty), which I attended to within 48 hours of receiving the kit. The second was a reminder from my GP to get some routine blood checks done, on my lipids and PSA (Prostatic Serum Antigen, the blood marker for prostate cancer), which I'd checked the year before. I impressed myself by getting the test done the next morning. I didn't think much about it, except that perhaps my lipids might be up a bit after some fancy dining during my recent travels. A few days later, (in early August) I was about to start seeing a list of my own patients, when I missed a call and my GP's receptionist left a message for me to make a non-urgent appointment. I felt a sudden jolt of concern, realising there must be something amiss. I focused on the patients I had to see, then returned the call. The next available appointment with my GP was in about three weeks. I didn't make any fuss, or hassle the receptionist, because I knew that I could look up my own results. Neither could I imagine waiting three weeks to find out, like most other people have to do.

Some lab reports highlight abnormal results in bold type or even red coloured font. As I opened the screen there were none of those bad signs, but there was some detail on the PSA report. It was still within the normal range, but at the upper limit; a year before it had been in the middle of the normal range, and the year before that, closer to the lower end of the range. So it had been steadily rising. There had been no relevant symptoms. This had simply been done as a screening test, and my GP was being efficient, organising regular follow ups.

There was, however, a component, the 'free fraction,' that was clearly abnormal, with an asterisk and comment suggesting this predicted a higher chance of neoplasia (cancer). I immediately assumed this had to be prostate cancer. (I wondered at the time how this would have played out had I not been a doctor with access to this information: one scenario could have been blissful ignorance for three more weeks; another could have been a high state of anxiety waiting to get in to be seen.)

I called a urologist and we had a frank and practical discussion. I arranged a formal referral to his office, and an MRI was ordered. I knew there was some debate about the pros and cons of prostate cancer screening, but it was not something that I'd kept up with. I was, however, familiar with some fantastic work done by Professor Rob

Newton, exercise physiologist at Edith Cowan University, on the role of exercise as an adjunctive therapy for prostate cancer. This was inspired by Rob's observations of his own father having surgery for prostate cancer and then being advised to rest. As he rested, he withered away, dying of a stroke less than two years after the prostate cancer was detected

So, once again I was in an MRI tunnel, this time looking at the other end of my body. Having completed the scan and dressing, the staff told me the radiologist could show me the results in 5 minutes. It suddenly struck me that in a few minutes I would learn about a whole new direction for my health. I wasn't afraid, but I did feel anxious; I think subconsciously I'd already assumed I had prostate cancer, but the implications had not yet sunk in. My radiology colleague led me to his work station to show me the scans. Despite never having seen a prostate MRI before, the glowing white dot in the right half of my prostate gland stood out glaringly, and I knew before he started to speak this was going to be bad news. I felt a welling up of emotion and didn't want to chat like a colleague when I was feeling like a patient. Once again, the limbo feeling of being both a doctor and patient was there, but this time without the advantage of the medical issues being within my field.

## 100 days of cancer

Two days later, Kirsten and I were looking at the same images on a big screen, this time with my medical school compatriot, a urologist specialising in prostate cancer. A huge torrent of information was presented to us, in a very positive and supportive way. We both liked his description of the situation as a 'speedbump in the road of your life journey.' We left with an impressive pack of information and a list of appointments with the various members of the team specialising in prostate cancer care. One thing I would like to have heard is a reminder that prostate cancer is one of the slowest growing forms of cancer, and so while we needed to get on and get this sorted out, the situation wasn't as urgent as any of the more rapidly growing cancers.

In addition to the comprehensive schedule of tests and appointments, I had other commitments to sort out. The Annual Scientific Meeting of the Stroke Society of Australasia was coming up in Melbourne in mid-August. I'd been looking forward to seeing my stroke colleagues face to face for the first time since COVID, and to present the data from our first human phase 1 study [24] of the neuroprotective peptide for Argenica Therapeutics. I was also scheduled to speak at the investigator meeting for the phase 2 study [25], which was coming together very nicely in a flurry of activity. It had been one of my career goals to help the scientists from the stroke research laboratory at the Perron Institute move the work from the laboratory into human studies. Now this was finally happening, I didn't want to miss this opportunity.

When I arrived at a cold and wet Melbourne airport late on a Tuesday afternoon, there was a message on my phone from the urologist. He confirmed what I had suspected, that this indeed was prostate cancer, with most of the specimens showing moderate to high grade change; as with the PD diagnosis, I had expected it, but it still hurt. The surgeon agreed to repeat the news and start formulating a plan during a three-way phone conversation with Kirsten. That was a tough and lonely night to be on the other side of the country, away from my wife.

I felt a great sense of frustration and exhaustion, as yet another health struggle now loomed. Looking back over the previous year or so, I'd now had COVID in May 2022, two cataract surgeries in August 2022, a depressive episode in September/October 2022 and deterioration of PD symptoms. By early 2023 it felt like I was starting to get back on top of things; then the retinal detachment in May 2023 knocked me down again. My vision was continuing to improve, but it was still obscured and I was resigned to the fact there were likely to be ongoing problems with my eyesight. And NOW CANCER!! I wondered if I had the energy left to go through another medical battle.

I looked out of the hotel room window at the Melbourne skyline. Unlike most hotel room windows, this one could be opened fully. For a very brief moment I looked down, wondering if I was high enough up to ensure certain death if I jumped. It was only a momentary thought, and I don't seriously think I would have ever acted on it, but it came up. I hope reading this is not distressing my family and friends; in fact, thinking of Kirsten and the boys was the main reason I quickly banished these dark thoughts. (I have included the issue of suicidal ideation in the aftermath of learning of bad medical news because I believe it is critical that doctors keep this in mind. Risk of suicide is particularly high after the diagnosis of degenerative neurological conditions.[26])

On my return to Perth I went straight from the airport to the urologist's office where I met with Kirsten, and then had a long appointment to explain the treatment options. Because of my relatively young age and otherwise reasonable health, as well as the absence of any obvious spread, a robot-assisted radical prostatectomy was recommended. My urologist was also in favour of adding pelvic lymph node clearance. I agreed and signed a consent form, with the date of surgery set for 20 September. I was particularly impressed that the surgeon had a supportive team whom I met over the weeks prior to surgery. This included the senior urology nurse, a physiotherapist specialising in pelvic floor strengthening exercises, and a sexual health nurse specialist. I was most impressed that there was also an exercise physiologist in the team. Kirsten and I had a valuable meeting with her before the surgery to outline a recovery exercise program, which included yoga, walking, strength and flexibility exercises, adapted to the surgery.

The next task was to speak to my family, friends and colleagues. Kirsten and I had learned a lot from disclosing the diagnosis of PD, particularly the emotional energy that was required. But this time, I was intrigued to observe a quite different reaction. When it became public knowledge that I had PD, people were very sympathetic, and almost intrigued that a neurologist should be affected by a condition from within their own specialty. Given the frequency of PD, I had never thought this to be particularly strange. (On reflection, I now think it says more about the undersupply of neurologists.)

In contrast, there was almost an indifference about my getting prostate cancer, especially among casual acquaintances, with a general attitude of 'lots of guys get this, you'll come through it fine.' (My family and close friends were much more understanding.) Strangely, the diagnosis made closing down my private practice a little easier. It sometimes felt like patients – and some colleagues – couldn't understand why I was finishing up clinical practice because of the slowness, fatigue and reduced confidence PD was causing me. On the other hand, the news that I had cancer, and was to undergo surgery on a set day, provided a clear reason and defined date.

Also, my own experience of the cancer diagnosis and my reaction was quite a contrast to that of the PD. I've often said the diagnosis of PD was almost a relief, and was no surprise. The prostate cancer was unexpected and sudden and had no symptoms, just the rising PSA, and the treatment made me feel terrible. Also, with PD, I had the advantage of already having a lot of knowledge, whereas with prostate cancer, I had only a little.

There was one more pleasant event before the prostate surgery: the Investiture Ceremony for presenting the King's Birthday Order of Australia honours at the Governor of Western Australia's residence. (I'd now known about my award, the Member of the Order of Australia, for nearly six months.) The presentation was highly organised and very formal; I was first up as the awards were presented alphabetically. The recipients had been taken aside half an hour before and had a dress rehearsal on the protocol. After my name was called, I stood and walked towards the governor while the announcer read a 30 second bio. It was a little distracting because the governor was shaking my hand and making conversation. Strangely, I didn't feel nervous at all. After the presentation there were photographs, mingling and tea. Most of the other recipients had multiple family members present, and I heard a few talking about heading out for celebratory dinners. It suddenly struck me that Kirsten and I were both not as revved up as most of the other attendees. Having been through the excitement of the WAOTY awards in June, we didn't have the energy to make this another big family event. However, the main reason for this feeling was that it was now a fortnight until the scheduled surgery. It was hard to believe that afternoon tea and awards with the governor were so quickly to be followed by cancer surgery – quite in keeping with the rollercoaster that was 2023.

The last few days before 20 September were nerve-wracking. I just wanted to hurry up and get it done. I had been thoroughly prepared by the excellent multi-disciplinary team and was doing extra sessions on my FIGHTMASTER boxing machine, and some extra weight work, knowing that these would be difficult to continue after the surgery. Another pre-operative challenge was to wean down my caffeine consumption. After my experience with a migraine after cataract surgery, I was eager to avoid a repeat. I had been a definite caffeine addict for more than thirty years, usually having two to four cups of black coffee and tea per day, along with more than 600 millilitres of diet Coke per day (and often much more than this). I was forever in a state where I was only a short step away from withdrawal, including headaches, lethargy and irritability. Surprisingly, the weaning process went smoothly.

I also wanted to minimise the risk of the terrible post-operative off state, like I'd had following the retinal surgery. The anaesthetist was very helpful, and came up with a plan to use a nasogastric tube to administer doses of soluble Madopar into my stomach at my routine time during the 4.5-hour operation, which included my usual 8 am and 11 am dose times.

The surgery took nearly five hours, and it was late afternoon before I was on the ward. That first night was tough; perhaps not quite as tough as the retinal detachment post-operative experience, but close. For about five hours, I had painful bladder spasms and nausea, which eventually subsided by about 9.30 pm.

Kirsten kindly roomed in with me on a fold up bed the first night; she was particularly vigilant to ensure I got my PD meds on time. The next couple of days were a challenge. At rest, I was reasonably comfortable, but any movement caused pain around the six small surgical wounds and the urinary catheter. I could feel the PD associated stiffness building as well. It also became apparent that a nerve in my pelvis (the obturator nerve) was not working, and had probably been stretched because of the posture and long time in surgery. This resulted in numbness in the inner part of my upper thigh, and weakness in several muscles that draw the thigh inwards. I realised this when some of the pains settled, and when trying to change my position in bed, found I couldn't move my left leg easily. In fact I later realised – with the help of the hospital physiotherapist– that I could only get my legs into and out of the bed by using a position where I didn't have to move my left thigh inwards against gravity. My left leg is my 'good leg,' not affected by PD, so I was very worried what this might mean for my future recovery.

On the second day after surgery I met the requirements to go home. As Kirsten pushed me in a wheelchair up the long corridor towards the hospital exit, I spotted a medical colleague walking towards us. I could see the expression of shock on his face when he saw me, washed out and frail and in a wheelchair. I told him how happy I was to be going home, and particularly pleased that I hadn't required his expertise as an intensive care specialist.

During the first week at home, Kirsten and I fell into a routine that we had planned with the exercise physiologist. This started with a short walk outside of about 100 metres, that felt like about 20 kilometres! There are several benches along the path around lake Gwelup, and my goal became to progress to the next bench, about another 100 metres away. The urologist had warned me I'd feel wiped out and initially would need two sleeps a day, and this was exactly right. I was surprised how solidly I could sleep in the late morning after the short, but exhausting walks. Pretty soon we added a second short walk in the afternoons and some gentle yoga, all under Kirsten's watchful eye.

Because I wasn't working or golfing, I found I now had the rare gift of some time on my hands, even though that was not combined with much energy. I watched more television than I ever have previously, and read copious amounts of fiction, mainly murder mysteries. My Kindle almost never left my side.

Eight days after the operation, the future became uncertain again. We were back in the surgeon's office for a check-up and review of the pathology. It was the classic good news and bad news scenario. The prostate cancer was all gone, with clear margins; this means there were no cancer cells at the edge of where the surgeon had removed tissue. There had, however, been involvement of two lymph nodes immediately next to the prostate. It made us all feel justified in undergoing the pelvic lymph node clearance component of the surgery and my surgeon gave a cautiously optimistic assessment. Re-testing of the PSA six weeks after the operation would provide more information. If that was undetectable, we could be reasonably assured of a cure. If it was detectable, there were several options to consider. In the meantime, the focus was on recovery and rehabilitation. I gradually increased the walking and Kirsten adjusted the yoga to focus on flexibility and balance. We worked closely with the exercise physiologist who provided great advice and oversight of the program. This included the addition of some resistance training using flexible bands, aimed at building up core strength without unduly straining the pelvis. There were also the ongoing pelvic floor exercises, to work on continence and management of bowels, and fluid intake to help with that. My caffeine intake now comprised about half a cup of hot black tea in the morning, taken to get my bowels moving. My previous coffee and Diet Coke consumption would have irritated my bladder and made my continence recovery much slower and more difficult.

Four weeks after the surgery I was able to walk a complete lap of one of the smaller loops around lake Gwelup. It was still difficult to walk, and I had to focus carefully on my posture and foot placement. Kirsten accompanied me for most of these walks, and was quick to correct me if I started to slouch forward or splay my feet out. I began to make a few trips to the golf course to practice; I had been putting in my front yard almost from the start (I admit I did a bit of putting while the urinary catheter was still in, just to see if I could!). I was pleasantly surprised to make reasonable contact with my first few shots, but was very careful to swing at only about 50% of usual effort because my lower abdomen was still quite uncomfortable when stretched.

The time for my cancer results arrived. The plan was for Kirsten and I to go to the appointment with the surgeon and hear the news together.

As the time drew nearer, I became anxious. Perhaps I was making too much of this, but I perceived it as a key juncture. The day finally came; 9 November 2023. As we walked into the surgeon's office, he handed me a piece of paper. It was the lab result:

PSA < 0.01; that is effectively zero!

Many patients are so overwhelmed at hearing bad news like 'you have PD' or 'you have cancer' that they don't take in what is said after that. What I hadn't realised was the same thing can happen with good news. What I do remember him saying was, 'David, you had cancer,' emphasising the 'had' as a past tense. Suddenly I felt a burden had been lifted. I would still need ongoing PSA checks, but for the first time in 2023 I felt I finally had some good news about my health. I'd learnt about the rising PSA on August the second. I realise that biologically, the cancer must have already been there for some time before, and there may be more issues yet to come, but 2 August to 9 November was 100 days; 100 days of cancer. That's more than enough for me!

## Fightback

The news of the zero PSA was a turning point. I felt I could start making plans again and look forward. More good news arrived in the form of an invitation from Dr Cormac Mehigan (whom I met at the Sixth World Parkinson's Congress in Barcelona) to play in the Irish Open Golf Championships for people with PD, to be held in early May 2024 at the Mt Juliet Course in County Kilkenny. This was excellent motivation for me to get back into good condition and return to golf. It also meant Kirsten and I could plan another trip to Europe; hopefully this time without COVID.

By the start of 2024 I was able to increase my exercise. I picked up my walking pace and with Kirsten's supervision, was doing yoga with relatively few modifications. I also spent a lot of time in our backyard swimming pool, doing specific exercises, working on my left leg to ward off possible muscle wasting from the nerve injury. By mid-January I was back using my home FIGHTMASTER machine, boxing training again. It felt great to be steadily improving. In February 2024, Rai started in-person boxing training sessions for the FIGHT-PD group in a small gym he'd set up in his garage. About half the participants in the trial got together again to train. Like me, most had been doing some training at home, but that is never as intense as in-person training, especially with Rai providing constant motivation. It was fantastic to see some of the FIGHT-PD team again. After just two one-hour sessions, I felt my energy levels were boosted. Within another month I was feeling terrific, and in better shape than I was prior to the prostate surgery. It was great to feel my strength and fitness improving again, at a rate I hadn't experienced since early 2020 when I was doing the initial training with Rai. Psychologically, it was a relief to know that, despite having PD, the ability to bounce back was still there. I was now a long way from how I had felt on that terrible lonely night in Melbourne after speaking with the urologist.

The goal of being well enough to travel to Ireland to play in the golf tournament was soon met, so we booked the trip. By April 2024, I'd been able to play several rounds at my local club without the use of a motorised cart. I actually felt much better walking the course, even though that required walking about 10 kilometres, including some infamously large hills. (The hill on the eighteenth has been dubbed 'cardiac hill' because of the number of angina attacks it has provoked.) I also played better when walking. I felt more connected to the course, and the walking kept my muscles warm, and ready to fire for the next shot. I started to use a technique the physiotherapists often apply to gait training in PD, namely making large, focused, deliberate movements, particularly of my right arm and leg. I found this helped me conquer those nasty hills without my leg failing. Just as the boxing posture is the antithesis of the pathological postures in PD, so sitting hunched into a golf cart exacerbates the problem – whereas walking counters it. Additionally, I'm sure it helped my swing. The large movements concept was originally used by speech pathologists to improve hypophonia (soft voice) in PD, by targeting use of a loud voice. The technique, LVST LOUD, is named for a patient, Lee Silverman who underwent the training with great benefit. It has since been modified for gait training (LVST BIG)[27]. The focus on making large movements increases speed in PwP, whereas focusing on speed of movements is less helpful. Given that speed is so important in the golf swing, this seemed like an ideal strategy for both walking and golf. On 10 April, the day before World Parkinson Day, I won a club competition for the first time in years. For a tantalising while I thought I was in with a chance of breaking par for the first time since the 1980s. This was not to be, but having the best handicap score by three shots in a field of 208 felt pretty good, and showed me that I'd come a huge way since the tough weeks after the prostate surgery. The fightback felt complete.

## Another trip

Our 2022 trip to Ireland and the UK was hampered by COVID and so the invitation to Ireland for the golf tournament provided a good chance to try again. In 2022, we missed out on time in Dublin, so we decided to start there before heading south to Mount Juliet estate for the inaugural Irish Open Parkinson's Golf Championship.

While at Mount Juliet, I was particularly reassured to see that people with much more disabling symptoms than I have, could still enjoy golf; this offered a positive glimpse of a possible future. Kirsten enjoyed the camaraderie and hospitality of the spouses, which was a terrific experience we hadn't really anticipated. I felt recharged and inspired. I was also reasonably happy to finish fourth. This was pleasing considering I was using hired clubs, and was much more familiar with playing on hard dry courses without thick, wet rough. I think most of the participants visiting from outside Ireland felt inspired to set up similar events in their home countries.

From there we flew to Copenhagen and spent more than a month travelling through Denmark, Norway and Sweden. We then spent the last few days in Barcelona, which we'd planned to visit in 2022. As is often the case when touring, we did a huge amount of walking, much of it on cobblestones and going up hills and mountains, and my body coped well with this. I was probably as tired at the end of a long day of touring as any other fifty-five year-old would be. To my surprise, I didn't feel the need for an early afternoon nap, as I often do at home. Also, thanks to the balance training from boxing and yoga, I averted several possible falls during our adventures. We returned to Perth in early June. Unlike in 2022, we returned fresh, and I was eager to work on some PD projects.

## Taking stock and seeing the silver lining

For the first time in two years I could assess where my PD was at without other conditions obscuring the picture.

Pre-diagnosis, my life was dominated by work. Thankfully, Kirsten kept me in check with Wednesday date nights, and I was playing golf fairly regularly. Without PD, perhaps I would have retired early anyway, played a lot of golf and travelled more. Perhaps I would have continued working too hard and had a stroke. Worse still, I could have continued in a sleep-deprived, caffeine dependent and moody state and made mistakes that harmed a patient. I am glad I recognised this and retired from acute stroke work when I did. In retrospect, the stress I put myself under during 2019 may well have worsened my PD. It wasn't until this contemplative time in 2024 that I came to fully appreciate that.

People unfamiliar with PD, and many PwP, may find it strange that I believe my life to be better for the experience of having PD. No doubt, my view might change in the future, but at this stage I feel as if I've been granted several surprising gifts: I have been forced to slow down and become more appreciative, and grateful of everything; I have come to understand the value of mindfulness and it has strengthened my already fantastic relationship with my wife. (Kirsten has been amazing with the 'in sickness' part of the marriage vows.) I have done things (like boxing training) and met people (like Rai) I never would have otherwise. Despite the physical limitations, I find myself to be mentally freer than ever before. I read much more widely now, including fiction. As a neurologist, it has given me an incredible opportunity to assist PwP and to help my colleagues understand more deeply the experience of living with PD. Also, I am grasping the chance to undertake several projects (see next chapter) that will keep me engaged in the field for as long as I like. I am not the only PwP to feel like this. In a 2022 paper[28], *The silver linings of Parkinson's disease*, the investigators conducted a survey utilising social media. They found that almost all respondents had some positive things to say regarding their experience of living with PD. Many aspects of their lives seemed to be improved, including better focus, improved coping skills, new activities, healthier lifestyle and improved relationships.

## Three PD projects

During the second half of 2024, three projects I had been working on all came nicely together. None of these were paid work, but have provided a great sense of satisfaction.

## Yoga for PD

Kirsten and I developed an 'introduction to yoga' course, supported by Parkinson's WA. The goal is to assess PwP thoroughly, assist with any necessary modifications, and give them the knowledge and confidence to attend regular yoga classes. My early and ongoing ineptitude with yoga provided Kirsten with ample opportunity to practice making PD-specific modifications over several years. In fact, this inspired her to undertake yoga teacher training. Just as in FIGHT-PD, I was a 'guinea pig' again, testing out postures and seeking those that might have the greatest benefit for PwP. Parkinson's WA provided funds for the yoga equipment and their PD nurse specialists helped select participants. Kirsten and I gained great satisfaction from doing this pro-bono, which also removed the complexities and stress that billing would require. We were fortunate to have free access to a large seminar room with a huge glass window overlooking a serene pond with gardens and birdlife; the perfect view for a yoga class.

The first class was in July 2024, in fact on my birthday. Friday morning quickly became my favourite time of the week. I would attend a boxing session with Rai and our PD boxing group at six in the morning, , then shower and go with Kirsten to the yoga class. It was eye opening for me to see Kirsten in full teaching mode and how amazing she is at communicating skills to people, and making adaptations where necessary. By the end of 2024 we had conducted two ten-week courses; the first starting with six participants and the second for four PwP. The small numbers enabled detailed, personalised instruction. At times, Kirsten became exuberant when those taking part could be seen making progress in their balance and movements. As with FIGHT-PD, a beautiful camaraderie developed among participants. In fact, towards the end of each series it was difficult to commence classes because there was so much chat going on! After a class, there would be further conversations over tea or coffee. These direct social interactions between PwP seem to be very important to them, and I suspect this has a positive impact on mental health.

We even wrote a short article[29]; 'Finding stillness: Introducing Yoga for People with Parkinson's Disease' published in *Journal of Yoga and Physiotherapy* in November 2024. In the article, we describe our personal experience with yoga, how it has helped both of us, how we developed the program and we also present some qualitative results. It was not an epic contribution to the PD literature, but it was a thrill to publish an article together.

In early December 2024, we both travelled to Shepparton, a major regional hub 180 kilometres northeast of Melbourne. A prominent geriatrician with expertise in PD, Arup Battacharaya, has hosted an annual meeting for PwP there since 2014. He contacted me in June 2024 and invited me to speak at the next meeting. I mentioned what Kirsten was doing with yoga and he immediately invited her as well. We were amazed that over 350 PwP, carers and healthcare professionals attended. In the morning, I spoke about communicating the diagnosis of PD, and during the afternoon session Kirsten presented what we'd done in the yoga program before leading the huge crowd in ten minutes of seated yoga. It was wonderful to have all those people quietly meditating at the end of the session. A delightful surprise awaited Kirsten when she finished. The annual general meeting of Parkinson's WA was held on the same day we attended the meeting in Shepparton;

Kirsten's efforts with the yoga program earned her the Parkinson's WA Volunteer of the Year award. Sheree Ambrosini, the lead PD specialist nurse from Parkinson's WA was also on the trip, speaking in the final time slot of the day. She announced Kirsten's much deserved award and presented her with a certificate.

## Support clinic for newly diagnosed PwP

In a collaboration with the Perron Institute and Parkinson's WA, I established a multi-disciplinary, nurse-lead group clinic for newly diagnosed PwP.

The main objective of this is to provide information and guidance during the first few weeks after the diagnosis, to find the best possible pathway to coping with PD, and optimising every aspect of help available. The time between the initial diagnosis visit and the first follow up with the practitioner can be extremely stressful. A huge number of questions arise and with increasing pressure on clinicians' time, it can be difficult to cover the many issues. A new PwP often leaves the consultation in a stunned state, usually forgetting what has been said after the words 'you have Parkinson's disease' have been spoken. They may be reticent to attend PD support groups, fearing interaction with others in a disabled state. Commonly, they turn to the internet and 'Dr Google.' They may be particularly vulnerable to disreputable information at this time. This is just one of the issues we address in this clinic.

The poster presentation[22] I gave at the World Parkinson's congress in Barcelona was a useful outline for shaping the structure of this clinic, and focused on the things that newly diagnosed PwP consistently say they want, such as quality, tailored information and time to ask questions. I spoke with several of the participants from FIGHT-PD about their experiences and what they felt could have been done to better support them around this time. The Parkinson's nurse specialists from the Perron Institute and Parkinson's WA, and a senior physiotherapist specialising in PD, collaborated in creating the draft structure of the clinic. We then presented this to the Movement

Disorder neurologists. After some minor tweaks, I presented to the general neurologists at one of the inter-hospital grand rounds, seeking their support and input. The final component of the clinic team, along with the nurses, physiotherapist and me, is our 'buddy system.' We created a roster of PwP who've had the diagnosis for several years and have been through the adjustment to the initial diagnosis phase. I select two of them to attend each clinic, some bringing their partners along, to share their experience and offer ongoing support to the new PwP.

Each clinic begins with introductions, then the nurses present some basic information about PD. The 'buddies' and I share our stories, and usually by then the new attendees are ready to talk and the questions keep on flowing. Some of the sessions have been quite intense, with emotional stories coming out. (The wife of one of the new PwP shocked the group when she described the turmoil they felt at diagnosis, so severe that when she left the consulting room she vomited.)

We provide written educational materials from Parkinson's WA, a list of physiotherapists with expertise in PD, information sheets for clinical trials and a document where I have collected the details of recommended books, websites, podcasts and videos. Most attendees will then be followed up by the Parkinson's WA specialist nurses. We hope this early contact and information helps newly diagnosed PwP to get through the difficult early weeks and also relieve some of the pressure on the nurses.

## Fazio's PD Fighters

Rai and his wife Bella, with some input from me, developed a series of instructional videos based on the FIGHT-PD study[22]. They included the warm up and the boxing rounds, with videos of Rai on the FIGHTMASTER machine, accompanied by written key points and safety issues. (We learnt that FIGHT couldn't be registered as a trade name, so a lot of work had to be done to remove it from the videos and documents, replacing it with 'Fazio's PD fighters'.) The plan was to use this as the basis to expand the program, making it available for use at home, or in a group setting. The full home package is a

FIGHTMASTER machine, a stand (like a music stand) on which to mount a video device (phone, iPad, laptop etc.,) and a custom floormat. The mat features lines and markings to enable correct foot positioning, based on what Rai and I had done with one of my old yoga mats. The videos can be accessed on line and build up from an introductory beginners' course to more advanced workouts.

This allows people to undertake the boxing program workouts from home with their own training machine. I am hopeful this will enable people living in the many geographically isolated regions of Australia (and elsewhere) to participate.

Rai had been running two in-person PD classes per week, where five of the original FIGHT-PD participants and a steady stream of new PwP trained at his home gym. Enquiries and requests to join had been steadily building for a couple of years and a bigger space was desperately needed. Rai had a long-term vision to create gyms at community centres where he could set up some FIGHTMASTER machines and run classes. His plan was to train boxing instructors to supervise classes where the instructional video would be played on a large screen behind the machines and which the instructors would use as the basis for workouts. Rai's wide sphere of contacts helped him gain the use of a room in the Loftus Community Centre in the city of Vincent – a densely populated inner- city region in Perth. The mayor and council generously allowed Rai to have three, two-hour timeslots per week within a large facility that included a twenty-four-hour gymnasium, the WA State gymnastics association, indoor basketball courts, a Pilates studio, coffee shop and numerous large rooms. The Perron Institute funded ten FIGHTMASTER machines and three large screen televisions. By early October, it was nearly ready to open. Rai arranged a practice run-through where nine PwP (including five from FIGHT-PD) and I did a work-out to test the set up. Channel 9 News filmed the whole session and then recorded interviews with Rai, myself and the mayor.

A public open day was held and was a huge success. I'd flown back from a stroke conference in Adelaide on the early flight that morning. The start was delayed by about fifteen minutes while we found extra chairs to accommodate more than 100 attendees. It was like a reunion, with many of my former patients and several of the PD yoga participants in the crowd. (It won't be long before there is a PwP who completes all three of the 2024 projects I am part of: The newly diagnosed clinic, yoga with Kirsten and boxing with Rai.) There was also the team from the Perron Institute newly diagnosed clinic, and CEO Stee Arnott. Travis Cruickshank, co-investigator of FIGHT–PD came along, and several people from Parkinson's WA were there. The delay was helpful, because I suddenly realised that Rai and I hadn't thought about what we were going to do for speeches. I quickly decided that I should speak after the mayor and then introduce Rai, following the principle of not following the 'main act.' Strangely, I didn't feel nervous while giving a short, unprepared public speech to a crowd buzzing with excitement. Rai then spoke from the heart, describing how the whole thing had evolved over about ten years, the last five with me. With the speeches over, the crowd could ask questions and then try out the equipment. About twenty PwP immediately signed up to attend. It was an amazing feeling to see Rai's vision coming together. Over the following weeks, Rai assessed the new recruits, dividing them into two groups according to level of mobility. By the start of December there were sixty PwP training regularly. I estimated this to be one of the biggest groups of PwP in the city, approximating or exceeding the size of many of the community PD support groups. I myself got back into training twice a week with Rai, on Monday nights and Friday mornings. It was great to see more PwP finally getting the benefit from the work we'd done over the past few years.

Meanwhile, Rai was mentoring other boxing coaches to prepare for expansion. The plan is to open another gym at Joondalup in the north, then Fremantle(south) and Midland (east). With time I hope it can expand even further.

## The future – fighting on

In addition to the three very satisfying projects that I hope can make an immediate difference to the lives of PwP, I have two longer-term and much bigger PD issues to work on. These are more like quests than projects, and will occupy me and many others for years to come. The first is the increasingly publicised issue of environmental toxin exposure and its relation to PD. The second addresses the idea that the way the initial diagnosis and early approach to PD is managed, may have an impact on the course of PD.

## Punching Paraquat

Having lived in rural regions of Western Australia from the ages of four till ten, I have long been curious about the possibility that exposure to herbicides or other substances may have been a factor in me developing PD. This interest intensified in late 2020 after I read the brilliant book[30], *Ending Parkinson's disease; A prescription for action* by Ray Dorsey, Todd Sherer, Michael Okun and Bastiaan Bloem. These are some of the most respected, and highly published medical and scientific experts in the world. Chapter two, 'A Man-Made Pandemic; how chemicals have fuelled the onslaught' gives an eye-opening rundown of the theory that the dramatic global increase in PD over the past twenty-five years is linked to environmental toxin exposure. In the final section of the book, they list '25 concrete steps we can and should take to reduce the worldwide toll of this daunting disease.' The first on the list is 'Ban paraquat and other harmful pesticides.' A report by the World Health Organization (WHO)[31] also lists this as their number one recommendation for prevention and risk reduction of PD.

Before describing my activities, beginning in 2021 and intensifying in 2024, to lobby for the banning of paraquat in Australia, here's a brief background.

Paraquat is a widely used herbicide that kills plants on contact by disrupting the photosynthesis mechanisms. It is highly effective in controlling weeds, including some that are resistant to other chemicals. In animals it has numerous detrimental effects at a cellular level, including damaging mitochondria[32], the important component of cells necessary for energy metabolism. There is no doubt that acutely, paraquat is highly toxic to humans. The US Environmental Protection Agency (EPA)[33] emphasises this - 'one sip can kill.' In fact, in some countries, most notably Korea, it has been widely used as a poison for suicide.[34] It is also a tragic cause of death by accidental ingestion, especially in Asia.[35]

For those wanting a concise review of the role of paraquat and other environmental toxins in PD, I can recommend 'Parkinson's Disease is Predominantly an Environmental Disease'[36], by Ray Dorsey and Bas Bloem in the *Journal of Parkinson's Disease*. It covers important issues regarding paraquat, such as its biochemical structural similarity to a toxin that is used to create animal models of PD; the findings of degeneration of dopamine cells in rats exposed to paraquat, and the epidemiological data finding an association between paraquat exposure and PD. It notes a 2011 study[37] of paraquat and rotenone which showed a 2.5-fold increased risk. It also mentions studies that suggest ongoing pesticide exposure after diagnosis may lead to faster progression of PD. I find this last point particularly worrying. As a result of concerns regarding both human and animal health and the environment, paraquat use has been banned in more than eighty countries worldwide.

However, it continues to be marketed and widely used in Australia, the United States, Argentina, Brazil and Japan. In Australia, some consider paraquat to be vital to the maintenance of crop yields and believe a ban would have serious impacts on global food supplies. There has been debate over many years regarding the reliability of the data regarding the long-term effects of previous and ongoing exposure to paraquat, and more specifically, its potential as a cause of PD.

It is because of this, that I 'entered the fray.'

In early 2021, the Australian Broadcasting Commission (ABC) ran a news story about paraquat and how 'one sip can kill.' I had not realised until then that paraquat was still being used in Australia, despite being banned in many other countries. I was also shocked to learn that the relevant regulatory body, the Australian Pesticides and Veterinary Medicines Authority (APVMA), had been reviewing paraquat since 1997. This motivated me to gather more information and fire off a letter to the APVMA in March 2021, in which I pointed out that the leading international experts who were the authors of *Ending Parkinson's Disease* were advocating a ban. The APVMA's response in April 2021 advised me that they 'consider all relevant scientific information when determining the likely risk before registering a product' and directed me to their 2016 report[38] which concluded 'that epidemiological studies do not demonstrate a robust statistical correlation between human exposure to pesticides, including paraquat, with Parkinson's disease.'

While I acknowledged the difficulties and complexity of the area, the response still got under my skin. Having stated they considered 'all scientific information,' their list of references seemed to be missing several important papers that were published before 2016. However, I was somewhat placated by the last sentence which advised that 'a full chemical review of paraquat' was currently underway, with a decision to be made by the end of 2021.

During the course of 2022 and 2023 I was distracted with the health problems that I described earlier, so I put the paraquat issue to the side for a while. When I re-emerged with renewed energy in early 2024, my interest was rekindled. I wrote earlier about my visit to Ireland in May 2024 where I played in the Irish Open Golf Championship for Parkinson's. During the second round we had to stand to one side while the grounds staff came by to spray the fairways, presumably with some sort of herbicide. The irony was not lost among our group of golfers with PD, all of whom (from three different countries) were aware and concerned about this issue.

I returned from that trip and began to look into things further. I was not surprised to learn that the APVMA review was still yet to be completed. The CEO of Parkinson's WA, Adjunct Professor Yasmin Naglazias was also very interested in the topic. She had noted the local Parkinson's support group in Albany, a major regional town on the south coast of Western Australia, was particularly large. We speculated this may be because many farmers retired from the dry harsh conditions of the wheatbelt to the cooler and more comfortable climate of the Albany region. In addition, one of my Western Australian colleagues had previously noted[39] what appeared to be a cluster of PD in a separate farming community in the state, and had suggested more evaluation be done. Yasmin and I decided this was long overdue, so we began exchanging ideas. We even met with a specialist occupational epidemiologist who had previously done some important work regarding the effects of asbestos exposure. These plans were put aside, however, because of two events that supercharged my interest in the topic.

The first, was the release of the APVMA's Paraquat Review Technical Report in July 2024. The other was a story about a cluster of PD amongst potato farmers in Victoria who had been exposed to paraquat, which aired on the Australian Broadcasting Commission (ABC) television program, *Landline* on September first. These two events became hot topics that towards the end of 2024 were to be vigorously debated in the Australian Federal Parliament[40,41].

The APVMA Paraquat Review Technical Report[42] is a 160-page document covering a wide range of issues. When I first saw it, I quickly focused on the section on neurotoxicity beginning on page 22, where there are several sentences discussing animal experiments with no references provided. This section concludes 'the overwhelming weight of evidence, is that paraquat does not induce neurotoxicity.' My initial reaction was that there must have been a typographic error and the 'not' shouldn't be there. The word 'overwhelming' certainly cannot apply because this is clearly not a one-sided issue, whichever way it is viewed. In a somewhat stunned state, I read on. Regarding human studies of occupational exposure, again statements are made without any detailing of references, concluding that 'the available epidemiology data is insufficient to conclude any association between paraquat exposure and neurotoxicity in the occupational environment.'

It took me some time to digest this. I carefully looked over the list of references. Two important meta-analyses[43,44] combining the results of dozens of studies and thousands of subjects, both published in 2019, were nowhere to be found. These both reported an increased risk of PD, with the usual cautions that must be made about finding associations not necessarily indicating causation.

More disturbingly, a pivotal paper[45] published in the February 2024 issue of the *International Journal of epidemiology*, 'Agricultural paraquat dichloride use and Parkinson's disease in California's Central Valley' by Kimberly C Paul and co-authors, was also not mentioned. The recall bias issue that had weakened some previous studies was overcome in this case because objective data was used. The investigators used data from the California Department of Pesticide Regulation, which is legally required to keep detailed information on commercial pesticide use. They were able to estimate paraquat exposure and relate that to residential and workplace addresses. Positive associations were found between exposure intensity, duration, and proximity of workplace to location to paraquat applications. I would have thought anyone following the field closely should have noted the importance of this paper.

The ABC *Landline* program showed farming families with multiple members with PD who had previously been exposed to paraquat. Dramatic black and white footage showed farmers standing in fields waving directions for the pilots of light aircraft, indicating where to drop their loads on the crops. It showed the spray drifting onto the farmers, who had no protective clothing or masks. Neurologist Associate Professor Wesley Thevasthan, was shown at a public information meeting for farmers giving a talk about the issue. Wes is a movement disorders specialist based in Melbourne and also has a farm in rural Victoria. His interest in the issue was sparked when he learnt paraquat was being used on a nearby property. The program also covered the controversy regarding the manufacturer of paraquat, Syngenta. There have been allegations that scientists working for Syngenta had found links between paraquat and PD but were prevented from revealing the data[46]. Additionally, it was alleged that Syngenta actively tried to discredit the work of independent researchers, particularly that of Professor Deborah Corey-Slechta, Professor of Environmental Medicine at the University of Rochester. She and her team focus on understanding the contribution of environmental exposures to human health.

The public reaction to the program was varied. On the one hand, there was quite justified empathy for the families who had been so tragically impacted and a sense of outrage that paraquat was still in use in Australia, admixed with the sense of anger that is stirred up by suggestions of big business conspiracy. Others, including some politicians and farming groups, heavily criticised the program, claiming it sensationalised the issue, and that showing footage of outdated practices (like the aerial crop dusting near farmers wearing no protective equipment) was a misrepresentation of current practices, and an over-dramatisation amounting to sensationalist journalism. The proponents of this view warned that paraquat was essential for effective farming, and removing it would have a dire impact on crop yields and threaten farmers' livelihoods.

Personally, this added to a sense of anger and injustice that I was already feeling after reading the APVMA report. I felt strangely energised by the prospect of taking up a worthy cause with the goal of reducing risk of PD. I found myself spending hours engrossed in the subject, making it a lead priority for my time. The APVMA was taking submissions from the public on the report until 30 October. I found myself focusing on preparing a much stronger effort than in my letter of 2021. It was pleasing to learn that I was not alone. Parkinson's Australia (PA) and another advocacy group, FIGHT-Parkinson's, were working rapidly to make a response – and PA was developing a lobbying strategy.

Meanwhile, my own plan was to garner support from the neurological community to back my submission, making it stronger than my solo effort in 2021. I'm not a great user of social media but for this, I made regular postings on LinkedIn trying to highlight the issue. Because Western Australia has only about forty active neurologists it's reasonably easy to contact them. About 80% of them are on a group e-mail list so I sent out an e-mail with an explanation of the situation, and a copy of the paper by Kimberly Paul[45]. I included a copy of the APVMA report (pointing out the findings regarding neurotoxicity on page 22), as well as a coversheet for a submission, if someone wished to make one themselves. I also included a link to the ABC *Landline* story. Meanwhile, Wes Thevathasan planned to do the same thing with his Victorian colleagues, and also pull together a literature review to include with his submission.

I was able to include a hot-off-the-press editorial by Bas Bloem[47] which gave an analysis of the Kimberley Paul paper. This was in early October, a few weeks before it appeared in the October issue of the *International Journal of Epidemiology*. I was extremely grateful for his rapid response and permission to use it for the greater good. The article explained how Kimberly Paul's study[45] was so important, particularly since it did not have the problem of recall bias which had weakened prior epidemiological studies. Bas and his co-workers also suggested that concerns regarding 'the safety of paraquat have become sufficiently large to invoke *the precautionary principle,*' where the safety of those working with pesticides and of residents living close to treated fields should be prioritised over crop yields and economic interests.

My key point was to recommend a collaboration between experts from the medical, agricultural and environmental areas to work towards phasing out paraquat, and for the government to support farmers to change their agricultural practices. I thus intended my submission to be a much deeper and more detailed suggestion of a pathway to change, rather than a simple 'ban paraquat.' To simplify things for my busy neurology colleagues, I suggested they return the e- mail with a simple 'yes' if they wished to support this. I also offered to speak to them directly. Then I contacted Australia's peak bodies for neurologists, the Australian and New Zealand Association of Neurologists, and the Movement Disorders Society of Australia and New Zealand, encouraging them the mail submissions. I was eager to get support from international leaders. I've mentioned previously my great respect for Bas Bloem and his amazing, broad PD research. He replied very quickly. I was also able to make contact with Ray Dorsey and Michael Okun from the USA. They kindly wrote directly to the APVMA. In addition, I received support from Professor Muhamed Salama from Cairo, who gave a platform address at the 2024 International Movement Disorders Society meeting on the topic of environmental toxin exposures and PD. The PD Avengers group in Canada also joined the list, thanks to their CEO Larry Gifford whom I had previously been in contact with regarding other PD issues. Larry has done some magnificent work assembling data regarding paraquat and PD.

I was interested to take a closer look at the people working at the front line with paraquat – farmers. I decided to go on a country road trip with my brother Mark and his wife Leanne, back to the small wheatbelt town of Pingaring, 260 kilometres east of Perth, where we had lived in the mid-1970s. The town was holding an event to commemorate the unveiling of a wall of plaques honouring the early settlers of the area. This provided a good reason for the journey, along with the additional motive to learn more about the use of paraquat. I wanted to find out if it was used in the paddocks surrounding the school and schoolhouse, as well as at the golf course where I had spent many hours practicing.. We left Perth on a Friday morning and drove to the southeast, and, after five hours reached Hyden; a small town famous for its fascinating geological formation, Wave Rock.

The next day we drove the 45 kilometres to Pingaring where we visited the farm of a primary school compatriot. The farmer kindly gave us a tour, showing us sheep shearing, fields and equipment, and giving us a rundown of cropping techniques. We learned that herbicides – including paraquat and glyphosate – are considered an integral part of the farming practice on this wheat and sheep farm and on many others in the area. Mark, Leanne and I were aghast to learn how glyphosate is sprayed directly onto canola crops as part of the cropping process. We saw several 1,000 litre containers of paraquat, and I also noted some smaller containers that were for other uses, but had 'paraquat' handwritten on them. Some of them were cracked and stained.

That afternoon we drove a kilometre up the road to the old school house, and then a little further to the golf course where we came across one of the locals whom we knew from all those years ago. We learnt that the golf course fairways were just mown, and not sprayed, because weeds made up most of the limited greenery. We then attended a function at the local town hall, attended by about 100 people, including many former residents returning for a visit. About a dozen had gone to the primary school when Mark and I were there. We had some very cautious discussions about herbicides. One of the farmers of my brother's age, with whom we'd kept up intermittent contact over the years, kindly offered to show us around his farm the next morning.

He showed us a canola crop with two invasive weed species attacking the edge of it. He also showed me some new machinery, designed for ploughing, digging up weed roots and destroying the weeds in one pass. He explained techniques that he used, and others that are on the horizon for minimising herbicide use. I was pleased to learn of his thorough knowledge of the issues and willingness to make changes, even though these added costs. His attitude was agreeably different to those of some of his colleagues with whom I'd been in contact prior to the trip. Some of them steadfastly refused to consider changing practice, claiming if paraquat and glyphosate were banned in Australia and the USA, this would reduce crop yields; combined with decreased grain production from the Ukraine, they feared this would trigger a global famine.

I had a lot to consider on the long journey back to Perth, along with some dozing in the back of my brother's car to catch up on sleep. The trip was inspirational, and gave me a deeper appreciation of the issues farmers faced. In a way, I slightly regretted supporting the call for a blanket ban, but the sight of the empty containers lying around, increased my concern for the farmers and their families who were at the front line of exposure. I concluded that even if I hadn't been exposed at the golf course, it was more than likely that paraquat was (and still is) used within metres of where I had lived and schooled for three years. I have always been careful not to state or assume that this was causative in my personal case, but I consider it may have made a contribution.

Upon returning to Perth, I set about finalising my submission to the APVMA.

Monday 28 October was the Parkinson's Australia National Day of Action to ban paraquat in Australia. It was a very busy time for me. ABC radio played a pre-recorded interview I had done with Andy Burns, the journalist who prepared the *Landline* story. This triggered four live radio interviews across the nation.

Following this day, there were plenty of supportive comments on line, and the Perron Institute received calls and e-mails from quite a mixed group of people. One was a concerned farmer who wanted to explain how he and many of his colleagues considered paraquat essential to their practice. Others wanted to share their concerns regarding prior exposure to paraquat. This included an amazing call from a man in Queensland who had worked in a plant nursery for more than ten years, using paraquat and other chemicals. He recalled having skin reactions, coughing fits and nausea after a session of spraying, while using only minimal personal protection. His boss was not particularly worried since he was under the impression that paraquat 'wasn't shown to have long term side effects.' The boss explained that the skin problem was just like a superficial burn, only affecting the outer layers and not going any deeper; he thought paraquat was much safer than the other herbicide glyphosate which, in his 'expert opinion' penetrated into the bones and caused cancer. The worker, who continued to plead for adequate protective equipment, was eventually able to leave this job, but is now chronically unwell and fearful for his future.

Just prior to Christmas 2024, the APVMA released a statement explaining that because of a high volume of submissions to the public consultation process, the final regulatory decision would be pushed back from the second to the fourth quarter of 2025. This delay is frustrating, and adds to the years of previous delays. I am, however, optimistic it may mean that the APVMA needs extra time to alter their position. At a bare minimum, I hope that the emerging data and opinions from experts in PD such as Ray Dorsey and Bas Bloem, will now be recognised by Australian regulators. However, a complete ban of paraquat and other toxic chemicals still seems to be out of reach for many members of the Australian agricultural industry. I plan to continue to press for collaboration between agricultural, medical and environmental experts to advance the issue. My view is that collaboration rather than confrontation will be the best way to move forward. Somehow, there has to be an alternative to using paraquat and similar toxins. This pathway needs to be carefully constructed, not 'bulldozed,' and there needs to be incentive to follow it.

A brilliant opportunity to do this arose when I learned about the 2025 Western Australian, Australian of the Year winner, awarded jointly to Ian and Dianne Haggerty. They have been leaders in ecologically friendly farming practices for over twenty years, successfully running sheep and grain producing farms in the Western Australia southern wheatbelt region using mulches, worms and other techniques to optimise the microbiome of the soil they are harvesting. Farmers from around the world have become interested in their work, which has virtually eliminated the use of herbicides and minimised the use of fertilisers.

What they are doing in the farming world aligns exactly with what I hope to achieve through this campaign against the use of paraquat. Their focus on improving the soil microbiome links beautifully with current ideas about the important role of the gut microbiome in the genesis of PD. We plan to further this collaboration during 2025, with the first step being for me to speak at the Parkinson's Australia national conference to be held in Canberra in April. This may provide an opportunity to get the message across to some federal politicians. The Haggertys' high profile in the farming community, coupled with their award, should help us to gain some ground. The fight against paraquat is one I feel very motivated to continue.

## Can the course of PD be altered? Studying the course of PD, and ways to favourably influence it

I believe that some of the current and older views on the course of PD may soon become outdated. These views paint a picture of relentless, inevitable decline at a linear rate. I suspect that is not the case, because the data on which they were based is probably inaccurate, and because I personally know numerous PwP where this just isn't true.

Up until recently, PD was a clinical diagnosis; that is, the core examination feature of bradykinesia (slow movement) accompanied by a resting tremor, rigidity, or both[48]. (A good response to L-dopa can add to certainty, and other mimics need to be ruled out.) Not surprisingly, these complexities and the inherent nuances of the neurological examination mean that the diagnosis can often be wrong. A review[49] of the literature suggested that the accuracy of clinical diagnosis, when compared with what was a 'gold standard' (usually pathological examination of the brain) was about 80%. The figure was a little higher (up to 84%) when made by experts in movement disorders, and as low as 74% with non-experts. Because of this inaccuracy of diagnosis, I am certain that much of the data on which prognosis and outcome in PD are based, include a substantial number of people who do not actually have PD, and also miss many people who do. I suspect that this results in the inclusion of patients who turn out to have one of the Parkinsonian syndromes like Lewy body dementia or multi-systems atrophy (MSA), which deteriorate more rapidly than PD. Also, those with very mild, early symptoms of PD may yet be diagnosed and are therefore not considered. The net effect of these two factors would be that the overall prognosis appears worse than it really is.

We are currently on the brink of having access to new diagnostic tools that allow for much more secure diagnosis and accurate prognostication.

In 2023, there was great excitement following the publication of a study[50] that described the utility of measuring alpha synuclein in the spinal fluid, and using that as a bio-marker to help diagnose the disease. A bio-marker is a measurable biological feature that may aid in the diagnosis, in some cases assess the severity, and ideally track the course of a condition. Tumour markers in the blood are an example, as illustrated in my own experience with prostate cancer and PSA. There continues to be a flurry of activity in this field with blood testing for alpha-synuclein and other potential biomarkers being developed. An international group of highly regarded experts in PD produced 'A Statement of the Movement Disorders Society (MDS) on Biological Definition, Staging and Classification of Parkinson's Disease'[51]. This cautions that there are still large knowledge gaps, and much work is yet to be done. My hope is that it helps to galvanise researchers and clinicians to work towards a more comprehensive understanding of PD. At a fundamental level, knowing with much more certainty that an individual actually has PD is obviously of huge importance. A further layer of information might be gained from genetic testing, where we already know that certain genetic abnormalities give rise to PD syndromes that carry a different prognosis to PD overall[52]. Using these tools, I hope that experts will soon be able to much more accurately forecast the course for each individual PwP and potentially tailor personalised treatments accordingly.

In addition to our models of PD being flawed, the perception that clinicians, general public and PwP have of what PD really is, may also be inaccurate.

In July 2020, Professor Michael Okun and his colleague Melissa Armstrong published a very important article in *JAMA Neurology*[53]: 'Time for a New Image of Parkinson Disease.' The article explains how the common perception of a PD patient is of an elderly, frail, white man, as sketched by the early English neurologist Sir William Gowers, way back in 1886. Such an image adds to stigma, fails to acknowledge the diversity of presentations across age, and gender and ignores how many with PD can continue to live active and meaningful lives. They hint that negative perceptions can feed into a self-fulfilling prophecy. I expanded on this in a comment on the article that was published in *JAMA Neurology*:

> I suspect that mental perception of PD may even influence progression; if a negative, nihilistic image is formed around the time of diagnosis, the self-fulfilling prophecy concept, combined with apathy, could contribute to lack of engagement in physical therapy and mobility, which I suspect accelerates progression.

It worries me enormously that if clinicians provide an overly bleak picture, or even if they don't and patients perceive a bleak picture, this might actually be worsening outcomes. Nonetheless, I strongly suspect that the course of PD can be favourably altered by the following combination of factors:

1. Early (within a month or two of diagnosis) provision of accurate, individually tailored information about PD combined with peer and psychological support.

2. Presentation of this information in a positive manner, encouraging individuals to take charge of their health.
3. Implementation of a comprehensive exercise program designed by professionals, which adapts to individual requirements and has flexibility to change according to intercurrent issues.
4. Ongoing multi-disciplinary, patient-centred support.
5. Attention to diet and lifestyle factors, including stress reduction.

Additionally, I think there is much to be learned from data that dissects the characteristics of those PwP who seem to have a more 'benign' course and who continue to live very well after decades of having PD. Recent work[54] using machine learning techniques to analyse data in the Parkinson's Progressive Markers Initiative (PPMI) study, identified three subtypes with distinct progression pattern: 'inching pace,' 'moderate pace' and 'rapid pace.' Differences in genetic profiles, and other factors, including the potential to benefit from drug therapies, are being actively explored with this method. Another approach is to compare those PwP who are doing well after a long period of time, with those who are not doing well. Even though these findings may not necessarily be definitive, the observations are very interesting. The prominent naturopath, Dr Laurie Mischley[55,56] is doing some fantastic work in the area, and also champions the idea that the course of PD can be favourably altered.

I still have much work to do to back up these ideas with solid data. Once collated, I aim to synthesise this data into an article to submit to a medical journal, and will continue to discuss the idea with PwP and medical colleagues. In the back of my mind is an embryonic plan to assemble a team of people who have similar views and write a short book.

# Finale (for now)

By December 2024 I had been on medications for PD for more than six years. I take fifteen tablets per day, carefully time my meals to optimise absorption of the tablets, and do some form of exercise every day. I've had some frightening glimpses of what I am like when I stray away from these fundamentals, especially when triggered by other medical conditions. For some time, I'd had the feeling that I was only just keeping on top of things, and that anytime soon there would be a deterioration. At the start of 2023, I felt I was likely heading towards DBS (deep brain stimulation) reasonably soon. Just over a year later, I realised I'd recovered to the point where I was prior to the prostate surgery, and was beginning to improve even further. This filled me with hope that I could remain well for longer than I had thought. However, somewhere from about September 2024, I felt I was going down again, with my right foot and leg becoming more troublesome with slowness, weakness and dystonia. For the first time, I began to experience an intermittent tremor in my left hand. I plan to further cut back on my work to enable me to focus on keeping well through exercise, attention to better sleeping patterns and some dietary changes. I hope to continue with the specific projects and 'quests' I've outlined. The slight deterioration has also encouraged me to complete this book while I am still well enough to endure the efforts required for publication.

I began writing this book around Christmas 2020; by Christmas 2024, I felt it was a good time to finish. I hope that my adventures might resonate with other PwP and my experiences help in some way. Additionally, I hope that my colleagues don't consider that I am being critical of their difficult work. It is my intention to continue to advocate for PwP from my curious position as a neurologist with PD, particularly in encouraging clinicians to communicate more freely and with a more positive outlook. A fantastic paper[57] 'Delivering the diagnosis of Parkinson's disease-setting the stage with hope and compassion,' published at the end of 2023 concludes with a statement I thoroughly endorse: *the time has come for cautious hope instead of conservative paternalism.*

I continue to have hope, for myself and the many other PwP, that there will be advances which can improve our lives, even if it is not a cure. In the meantime, I intend to fight on.

David Blacker

January 2025

***Special note**

I mentioned Peter Coghlan in the section *2023 – a rollercoaster of events*. I must acknowledge Peter as a wonderful role model for fighting a neurological disorder. In 2011 at the age of thirty-one, he suffered one of the most disabling kinds of stroke, resulting in the 'locked in syndrome' (LIS) where virtually all muscles of the body, except for breathing, are paralysed. Typically, only the eyelids can move, along with some flickers of the eye-lids and face. If not complete, there can also be tiny voluntary movements in the limbs. In many patients the only way to communicate is by blinking. I became his neurologist after the acute phase of the stroke was over, when decisions about rehabilitation were required. I recognised there was some potential for recovery and gained the impression he was a very determined individual. He proved this during inpatient rehabilitation under my team at the Royal Perth Rehabilitation Hospital. After six months of intensive therapy and Peter spending virtually every waking moment focusing on regaining control of his body, he was able to walk. The improvements continued well after discharge. Just two years after the stroke, Peter and I walked the 12-kilometre Perth City to Surf event together. He went on to write an inspirational book about his experiences, *In the blink of an eye; reborn*. I was honoured to be asked to write the foreword to Peter's book. I still see Peter intermittently, and have done some boxing training with him; he now has a FIGHTMASTER machine. His journey, and the privilege I have had in being a small part of it, has helped inspire me in my own FIGHT with PD.

# Acknowledgments

The first acknowledgment must be to Kirsten; without her love and care I could not have written this book. In fact, without her efforts I might not even be able to walk now. With admirable self-control she left me with the space to make this very much my version of the path we are taking together. PD affects the whole family, so I must thank my sons, James and Matthew for their support. My father, Kevin has seen my mother, Cynthia develop Alzheimer's disease about the same time I've had PD. I'm further motivated to keep well for their sake.

There are many other PwP who I consider friends who have given me strength and encouragement over these last few years, and provided me with the inspiration to share my experience. There are several colleagues who have provided me with excellent medical care for PD and my other health challenges during this time. I spent some time deciding on which of my neurological colleagues to consult. Dr Wally Knezevic has been an excellent choice.

With respect to the writing and publishing process, I have found the Australian Society of Authors to be an invaluable resource. I must thank my neighbour, Brooke Johns for putting me in contact with Ian Hooper at Book Reality. Ian's skills and knowledge have indeed made this book a reality.

# About the Author

David Blacker AM, MB BS, FRACP's career in medicine and neurology has spanned four decades, during which he helped lead a revolution in the care of acute stroke. As a doctor, mentor and medical researcher his work has impacted many thousands of patients, hundreds of doctors and numerous scientific medical fields.

In 2018 he received the life changing diagnosis of Parkinson disease, which lead to a reshaping of his career to focus on research and advocacy in PD. He now writes and speaks widely about his personal experience with PD, and hopes to assist others by sharing this. Additionally, he is striving to help his medical colleagues gain a greater insight into living with PD and to improve their communication and interactions with people with PD.

This change in direction created some unexpected opportunities, such as the surprising collaboration with former national boxing champion, Rai Fazio to develop a boxing exercise program for PD. This included a ground breaking clinical trial (FIGHT-PD) and now highly successful training program which is improving the quality of life for people with PD.

In 2023, he faced further challenges with complications following prostate cancer surgery, and a retinal detachment leading to impaired vision. Using the knowledge gained through exercise based therapy, and with the expertise of his wife Kirsten, in yoga, he has fought back to become fitter than ever. This journey from being a doctor to a patient, and all the challenges that posed are described in, *My FIGHT with PD, a neurologist with Parkinson disease*.

After retiring from clinical practice in 2023, he has continued research into PD and stroke, based at the Perron Institute for neurological and translational science. Also in 2023, he was awarded a membership of the Order of Australia (AM) for his service to medicine and neurological research.

# References

[1] Ayesu K, Nguyen B, Harris S, Carlan S. The case for consistent use of medical eponyms by eliminating possessive forms. Journal of the Medical Library Association 2018.

[2] Lees A, Hardie R, Stern G. Kinesogenic foot dystonia as a presenting feature of Parkinson's disease. *J Neurol Neurosurg Psychiatry* 1984;47:885.

[3] Thickbroom G, Byrnes M, Blacker D, Morris I, Mastaglia F. A functional MRI protocol for localizing language comprehension in the human brain. *Brain Research Protocols*. 2003;10:175- 80.

[4] Blacker DJ. A neurologist with Parkinson disease. *Practical Neurology* 2020;0:1-2.

[5] Ridgel A, Vitek J, Alberts J. Forced, Not Voluntary, Exercise Improves Motor Function in Parkinson's Disease Patients. Neurorehabilitation and Neural Repair. 2009, Vol 23 (6) 600-608.

[6] Fuzhong L, Harmer P, Fitzgerald H et al. Tai Chi and Postural Stability in Patients with Parkinson's Disease. *N Eng J Med* 2012;366:511-519.

[7] Morris M, Ellis T, Jazayeri D, Heng H, Thomson A, Balasundaram A, Slade S. Boxing for Parkinson's Disease: Has Implementation Accelerated Beyond Current Evidence? *Front Neurol*. December 2019. 10:1222.

[8] Combs S, Diehl M, Staples W, Conn L, Davis K, Lewis N, Schaneman K. Boxing Training for Patients With Parkinson Disease: A Case Series. *Physical Therapy*. 2011 Vol 91 (1) 132-142.

[9] Combs S, Diehl M, Chrzastowski C, Didrick N, McCoin B, Mox N, Staples W, Wayman J. Community-based group exercise for persons with Parkinson disease: A randomized controlled trial. *Neurorehabilitation* 2013, 32: 117-124.

[10] American College of Sports Medicine. ACSM's guideline for exercise testing and prescription. Lippincott Williams & Wilkins; 2013: Mar 4.

[11] Domingos J, Radder D, Riggare S, Godhino C, Dean J, Graziano M, de Vries N, Ferrreira J, Bloem B. Implementation of a Community-Based Exercise Program for Parkinson Patients: Using Boxing as an Example. *Journal of Parkinson's Disease* 2019. 9:615-623.

[12] Schenkman M et al. Effect of High-Intensity Treadmill Exercise on Motor Symptoms in Patients With De Novo Parkinson Disease. *JAMA Neurology*. 2018;75 (2):219-226.

[13] Van der Kolke N, de Vries N, Kessels R, Joosten H, Zwinderman A, Post B, Bloem B. Effectiveness of home-based and remotely supervised aerobic exercise in Parkinson's disease: a double-blind, randomized controlled trial. *Lancet Neurology*. 2109;18:998-1008.

14 Mak M, Wong-Yu I. Six-Month Community-Based Brisk Walking and Balance Exercise Alleviates Motor Symptoms and Promotes Functions in People with Parkinson's Disease' A Randomized Controlled Trial. Journal of Parkinson's Disease. 2021. 1431-1441.

15 Borg G. Borg's perceived exertion and pain scales. *Human Kinetics* 1998.

16 De Freitas T, Leite P, Dona F, Pompeu J, Swarowsky A, Torriani-Pasin C. The effects of dual task gait and balance training in Parkinson's disease: a systematic review. *Physiother Theor Pract* 2020;36(10):1088-1096.

17 Blacker D, Fazio R, Tucak C, Beranek P, Pollard C, Shelley T, Rajandran S, Holbeche G, Turner M, Cruickshank T. FIGHT-PD: A feasibility study of periodized boxing training for Parkinson disease. *PM&R* 20231-11.

18 Reijinders J, Ehrt U, Weber E et al. A systematic review of prevalence studies of depression in Parkinson's disease. *Mov Disorders* 2008;23:183-189.

19 Perez-Torre P, Lopez-Sendon J, Barral V, Parees I, Fanjul-Arbos S, Monreal E, Alonso-Canovas A, Castrillo J. Concomitant treatment with safinamide and anti-depressant drugs: safety data from real clinical practice. *Neurologia (Engl Ed)* 2021 Sep 10.

20 Johnson S, Davis M, Kaltenboeck A, Birnbaum H, Grubb E, Tarrants M, Siderowf A. Early retirement and income loss in patients with early and advanced Parkinson's disease. *Appl Health Econ Health Policy* 2011;9 (6): 367-376.

21 Saver JL. Time is brain-Quantified. *Stroke* 2006;37:1; 263-266.

22 Blacker D. A neurologist with PD: What I've learnt about being a patient and person with PD. Abstracts of the 6th World Parkinson Congress, July 4–7 2023 Barcelona, Spain. *J of Parkinson's Disease*, vol 13, no. S1 p349.

23 Shrag A, Modi S, Hotham S, Meritt R, Khan K, Graham L. Patient experiences of receiving a diagnosis of Parkinson's disease. *Journal of Neurology* 2018;265: 1151-1157.

24 Blacker DJ, Redfern A, Thomas M, South S, Knuckey N, Meloni B. A phase 1, double-blind, randomized, placebo-controlled, sequential-group study to assess the safety, tolerability and pharmacokinetics of single ascending doses of ARG-007 in healthy participants. *Int J of Stroke* 2023, Vol. 18 (2S) 1.

25 Blacker DJ, Hankey GJ, Thomas M, Phillips T, Bailey P, Donnan G, Saver JL, South S, Knuckey N, Meloni B. Phase II, double-blinded, randomized, placebo-controlled study to determine the safety, preliminary efficacy and pharmacokinetics of ARG-007 in acute ischaemic stroke patients (SEANCON). *Int J of Stroke* 2023, Vol. 18 (2S) 46.

26 Nafilyan V, Morgan J, Mais D, Sleeman K, Butt A, Ward I, Tucker J, Appleby L, Glickman M. Risk of suicide after a diagnosis of severe physical health conditions: A retrospective cohort study of 47 million people. *The Lancet Regional Health-Europe.* Vol 25 February 2023.

27 Fox C, Ebersbach G, Ramig L, Sapir S. LVST LOUD and LVST BIG: Behavioral Treatment Programs for Speech and Body Movement in Parkinson Disease. *Parkinson's Disease* Volume 2012, Article ID 391946.

28 Alonso-Canovas A, Voeten J, Thomas O, Gifford L, Stamford A, Bloem B. The silver linings of Parkinson's disease. *npj Parkinson's Disease* (2022)8:21.

29 Blacker DJ, Blacker KM. Finding Stillness: Introducing Yoga for People with Parkinson's Disease. *Journal of Yoga and Physiotherapy.*

[30] Dorsey R, Sherer T, Okun MS, Bloem BR. *Ending Parkinson's Disease. A prescription for action.* March 2020

[31] Parkinson disease: a public health approach: technical brief. World Health Organization; 14 June 2022.

[32] Costantini P, Petronilli V, Colanna R, Bernardi P. On the effects of paraquat on isolated mitochondria. *Toxicology 1995*, vol 99; 77-88.

[33] https://www.epa.gov/pesticide-worker-safety/paraquat-dichloride-one-sip-can-kill accessed 30th December, 2024

[34] Seok S, Gil H, Jeong D, Yang J, Lee e, Hong S. Paraquat intoxication in subjects who attempt suicide: why they chose paraquat. *Korean J Intern Med* 2009;24:247-251.

[35] Gawarammana I, Buckley NA. Medical management of paraquat poisoning. *Br J Clin Pharamcol* 2011;72:745-757.

[36] Dorsey ER, Bloem BR. Parkinson's Disease is Predominantly an Environmental Disease. Journal of Parkinson's Disease 2024;14:451-465.

[37] Barbeau A, Dallaire L, Buu NT, Poirier J, Rucinska E. Comparative behavioural, biochemical and pigmentary effects of MPTP, MPP+ and paraquat in Rana pipiens. *Life Sci* 1985, 37, 1529-1538.

[38] Australian Pesticides and Veterinary Medicines Authority. Paraquat toxicology report- supplement II neurotoxicology. October 26th, 2016.

[39] Panegyres PK, Gray V, Barrett L, Perceval S. Neurological disorders in a rural Western Australian population. *Internal Medicine Journal* 2010;40:209-213.

[40] Hansard Commonwealth of Australia parliamentary debates. House of Representatives Private Members' Bill . Pesticides speech, Webster Anne MP, Monday 4th November 2024.

[41] Hansard Commonwealth of Australia parliamentary debates. Communications Legislation Amendment (Combatting Misinformation and Disinformation) Bill 2024 second reading, Webster Anne MP, Wednesday 6th November 2024.

[42] Australian Pesticides and Veterinary Medicines Authority. Paraquat Review Technical Report. 30th July, 2024.

[43] Tangamornsuksan W, Lohitnavy O, Sruamsiri R, Chaiyakunapruk N, Norman SC, Reisfeld B, et al. Paraquat exposure and Parkinson's disease: A systematic review and meta-analysis. *Arch Environ Occup Health.* 2019;74(5):225-38.

[44] Vaccari C, El Dib R, Gomaa H, Lopes LC, de Camargo JL. Paraquat and Parkinson's disease: a systematic review and meta-analysis of observational studies. *J Toxicol Environ Health B Crit Rev* 2019;22:172-202.

[45] Paul KC, Cockburn M, Gong Y, Bronstein J, Ritz B. Agricultural paraquat dischloride use and Parkinson's disease in California's Central Valley. Int J Epidemiol. 2024;53(1).

[46] Carey Gillam AU, Secret files suggest chemical giant feared Weedkiller's link to Parkinson's disease. https://www.thwguardian.com/us-news/2022/oct/20/syngenta-weedkiller-pesticicde-parkinsons-disese-paraquat-documents

[47] Darweesh SKL, Vermueulen RCH, Bloem BR. Paraquat and Parkinson's disease: has the burden of proof shifted? *Int J Epidemiol* 2024;53(5).

[48] Bloem B, Okun M, Klein C. Parkinson's disease. *Lancet.* Published on line April 10, 2021.

[49] Rizzo O, et al. Accuracy of clinical diagnosis of Parkinson's disease: A systematic review and meta-analysis. *Neurology* 2018. 86(6):566-567.

[50] Siderowf A, Concha-Marambio L, Lafontant DE, et al. Assessment of heterogeneity among participants in the Parkinson's Progression Markers Initiative cohort using α-synuclein seed amplification: a cross-sectional study. Lancet Neurol 2023;22(5):407-417. (In eng). DOI: 10.1016/s1474-3.

[51] Cardoso F, Goetz C, Mestra A et l. A Statement of the MDS on Biological Definition, Staging, and Classification of Parkinson's Disease. *Movement Disorders* 2024, Vol 39, No 2.

[52] Aasly J. Long-Term Outcome of Genetic Parkinson's Disease. *J Mov Disord* 2020;13(2):81-96.

[53] Armstrong M, Okun M. Time for a New Image of Parkinson Disease *JAMA Neurology* 2020;77(11):1345-1346.

[54] Su C, Houi Y, Xu J, et al. Identification of Parkinson's disease PACE subtypes and repurposing treatments through integrative analysis of multi-modal data. *NPJ Digital Medicine* (2024)7:184.

[55] Fox D, Park S, Mischley L. Comparison of the Associations between MIND and Mediterranean Diet Scores with Patient-Reported Outcomes in Parkinson's Disease. *Nutrients*. 2022 Dec 6:14(23):5185.

[56] Mischley L, Lau R, Weis N. Use of a self-rating scale of the nature and severity of symptoms in Parkinson's Disease (PRO-PD): Correlation with quality of life and existing scales of disease severity. *NPJ Parkinson's disease.*(2017).

[57] Subramanian I, Pushparatnam K, McDaniles B, Mathur S, Post B, Schrag A. Delivering the diagnosis of Parkinson's disease - setting the stage with hope and compassion. *Parkinsonism and Related Disorders*. 118(2024)

www.ingramcontent.com/pod-product-compliance
Lightning Source LLC
Chambersburg PA
CBHW061232070526
44584CB00030B/4088